THAT
DIRTY FAT

A Guide
to Reducing
Body Toxins

By
Michael Hobson, D.C.

Copyright © 1994 Woodland Publishing, Inc.

Published By
Woodland Publishing, Inc.

Printed in the United States of America

Table of Contents

Readers Note: The first two chapters have scientific
                 references for documentation purposes
                 and to satisfy the very serious readers.

THAT DIRTY FAT

Accumulating and Reducing Body Toxins
The man made epidemic of the 20th Century

by Dr. Michael K. Hobson

PREFACE

This book is dedicated to the many millions who are suffering from environmental illness, knowingly or unknowingly. It has been written for those who suffer needlessly; for those who do not know where to turn for answers. This book offers the hope for their confusing, frustrating, and diverse symptoms.

The information contained in this book could help overweight people obtain effective and permanent weight loss. The following pages will provide hope, inspiration, and most of all, answers.

This is a book of objectives and a book of methods, a book that helps to clarify the effects of environmental illness and offers understanding and knowledge to the average person. With this knowledge, the patient can actively participate in his/her care and effectively overcome the causes of this modern-day malady.

I am dedicated, as a doctor and as a member of this human race, to research and to provide answers to health problems that could be avoided and eliminated, if the right information were available. The needless suffering of many with this illness could end if this knowledge would be applied to each individuals' life. There is no subject of greater physiological importance, in my mind, than the subject presented in the following pages. The welfare of each of us depends on the maintenance of physical health, and the elimination of toxins from our environment; particularly from our food. I offer this information with this assertion and conclude that these pages have certain value to all.

Chapter One

THE DISCOVERY OF BIOACCUMULATION

In the summer of 1986, Clark, a 51 year old male, entered my office desperately seeking help. His wife claimed that his condition was a very debilitating problem. When I first saw Clark, his face appeared abnormally red. When I asked why, his wife told me that it was a hypersensitivity to sun light from the medication he was taking. Due to Clark's mental confusion and depression, he was initially referred to a clinical psychologist and prescribed antidepressants, sleeping pills and phycotropic medications to stabilize his mood swings. Clark couldn't really communicate effectively during the initial five to eight visits over several weeks.

His wife informed me that he had been working with his son in Las Vegas doing construction work up until four months earlier. She related how Clark had always been very competent as a foreman due to his years of experience in all stages of construction. However, the last four to five months on the job, Clark started to become more and more disoriented and mentally incapacitated. The month before he had to quit, Clark couldn't read floor plans, couldn't understand directions given to him, and would make many mistakes. Finally his son, who was the owner of the company, had to let his own father go because of safety reasons.

Clark has been suffering frequent headaches, which I felt confident could be treated and eliminated with the usual spinal rehabilitation therapy. I recognized his other symptoms as relating to neurological system disfunction, and since I had some experience in this area, I prescribed the treatment that had been effective with this type of disorder. I prescribed a radical change in his diet, frequent exercise, and a regimen of pure water intake, consisting of one gallon daily.

I had always known since my days as an intern that diet was an extremely powerful tool for healing. I had also learned early on in my career that exercise naturally stimulated all body systems, including nervous and immune systems. And I felt that a high intake of pure water would help flush toxins and adequately hydrate the body.

After approximately two weeks of therapy, Clark began to show good signs of improvement. He was actually talking to me during visits in a rational and cognizant manner. His wife claimed he wasn't as depressed and was beginning to do things around the house. Clark claimed that he could concentrate better and make decisions. And his headaches were almost gone.

After about four weeks, Clark claimed to feel 80 to 90% improved and wanted to return to work. I instructed him to continue to eat, exercise, and drink water as prescribed.

He was able to successfully return to work and perform his job as before, without feeling like he was in a mental fog all of the time.

After my experience with Clark, I began to take a closer look at my clinical practice. I wanted to understand more about what caused Clark to become ill and why he improved. I had several working theories. But I wanted to know if there was anything necessary to improve, rehabilitate or strengthen my patients health, provided it fell within my scope of practice laws. I also decided that holistic medicine was the most logical approach to health care. Which means looking at the entire body and all of the related body systems as they relate to health and disease. Then finding natural methods of disease prevention, and the restoration of lost health is the next step.

Mainstream Chiropractic medicine teaches holistic health care dealing with spinal disease, injury, or disfunction. It also spends years teaching the chiropractic student principles of nutrition, biochemistry, biomechanics of the human body, pathology and other related diagnostic and treatment methods. Yet when a patient like Clark comes along, I didn't feel adequately prepared to deal with this type of complicated case.

After years of clinical practice, a doctor begins to develop an intuitive sense about his patient care. I had been treating patients for about four or five years, when I realized that something vital was missing. That quality holistic health care wasn't being offered to my patients, and I was determined to research and study, until I felt confident in this area and could effectively counsel my patients. It was at this time that I began my search.

In the fall of 1986, my diagnostic skills continued to be challenged by several other new patients who came in with a combination of symptoms that I felt uncomfortable treating. These symptoms included three or more of the following, which were recurrent or continuous in nature: Irritability, cold or flu-like symptoms, chronic fatigue, headaches, skin disorders, musculoskeletal pains, and increased irritations to dust or pollens. There were many seemingly unrelated symptoms in varied combinations that challenged me further yet inspired greater determination to find the answers. The normal diagnosis for this array of strange symptoms is often psychosomatic, but I was convinced that my patients were truly suffering from physiological illness.

Our professors taught us in chiropractic college to effectively deal with spinal disease or disfunction, and they taught us how to improve health through nutritional modifications, exercise and attitude. They also taught us when to refer to other practitioners in cases of advanced disease or something outside our scope of practice. I was faced with the challenge of helping those who had tried every other method and were looking to me for answers. They knew their symptoms were not psychosomatic, and having been to other doctors, felt anxious to find the help they needed. Since I was known for my success in effectively treating Candida, many of these patients with similar symptoms, were anxious to try what I prescribed.

In researching Candida Albicans Virus, Ebstein Barr Virus, Mononucleosis Virus, and several other illnesses, I began to realize that there was at least some common thread of apparent immune system disfunction or impairment. At this particular time, I was using a simple candida diet and educating patients about the cause, nature, treatment and prevention of the condition. I was also attempting to do therapy to strengthen the immune system. Some of my patients I was able to help, however some I could not, and I soon realized that there were further implications. There was a deeper or hidden cause, yet undiscovered.

It was around this time that I was lucky enough to meet an eccentric fellow (who's name I won't mention), whom I thought at the time was a little crazy. He related some information that both frightened me and yet fascinated me at the same time. I wasn't sure how much of this new information to believe, so I inquired as to his sources. He provided me with several research groups and federal agencies that I could contact, as resource information. Because of my inquisitive nature and desire to help suffering patients, I made a number of initial contacts and acquired some fascinating information.

The following information is a basic chronology of my personal discovery of bioaccumulation. It is included in some detail for the purpose of properly educating those who may be suffering with this condition. I have maintained that the more knowledge a patient has about his/her condition, the more equipped he/she is to participate in the cure. This knowledge motivates action and maintains persistence in treatment. It provides confidence in therapy, and keeps the patient from being influenced by well-meaning friends, or doctors.

One of the first pieces of research material I acquired was the EPA's FY82 NHATS study.(1) This particular study is the EPA's National Human Adipose Tissue Survey (NHATS), the nation's longest running program for monitoring human exposure to potentially toxic substances that persist in the environment. The study has been an ongoing program in one form or another since 1967, which monitors fat-stored substances in the human body to assess the chemical risk to the U.S. population. For many years, cooperating pathologists across the country have collected and shipped the necessary fat samples to OTS, (Office of Toxic Substances), in the Midwest Research Institute in Kansas City, Missouri. Many of these fat-stored substances commonly found in U.S. citizens are known human carcinogens, cancer causing, or in other words, lethal.

There are over 50,000 environmental chemicals with undetermined toxicity to investigate, and the NHATS program capacity can only deal with 12 or so a year. I soon discovered that we are left with many unanswered questions about just how much our environment is affecting us.

However, with this study, a number of now answered questions are yet producing many other serious health concerns. For example, the FY82 study concluded that 100% of the U.S. population are housing, in permanent storage in their fat, many known carcinogens. These are referred to as lipophilic toxins or poisons which are attracted to and absorbed by fats throughout the body. Many of these toxins, or bio-accumulations as they are often referred to, are absorbed into the various fats and other tissues of our bodies and remain there for many years causing untold damage to our health.

PCB's or Polychlorinated Biphenyls for example, bio-accumulate in human tissue and the levels increase as one ages.(2) Virtually all persons in the U.S. have some PCB in their bodies: the average 160 lb. male has a total body burden of 20 to 50 mg. PCB with approximately 1 ppm in fat.

The next questions one might ask are, "How are these toxins getting into our bodies, and how are these toxins affecting our health?" These are extremely important questions, and the beginning of understanding the bio-accumulation epidemic.

Until 1977, various U.S. companies produced many millions of pounds of PCBs. In fact, millions of pounds are still in place in closed systems in the U.S.. Until the mid 60's scientists didn't really know of the danger posed by PCBs. The stability properties of low water solubility, good insulating properties, high boiling points and resistance to chemicals that made PCBs so useful in industry, have allowed them to persist in our environment. Disposal of this deadly chemical compound into water and soil has led to the concentration of this compound, and others, into sewage, vegetation, marine life, and eventually humans (the top of the food chain). Therefore, we humans eat, breath and drink it. This and many other compounds are all around us, and it is just about impossible not to ingest, in one form or another, living in modern civilization.

To gain a little better understanding of how this man-made chemical compound affects our health, let's take a look at some of the disasters that have occurred in history where high levels were accidentally ingested by people. In 1968 an outbreak of PCB poisoning occurred in Japan. The disease was called Yusho which means "the oil disease." Yusho arose from ingesting rice oil contaminated with PCB-heat transfer oil. The average Yusho patient had eaten about 2 g of PCBs and a dose-response relationship was evident, i.e., the more PCB oil consumed, the more severe the clinical illness.

Yusho victims exhibited a latent period between ingestion of the oil and outset of symptoms. It averaged 71 days and ranged from 20 to 190 days. By 1978 a total of 22 deaths occurred among 120 of the Yusho victims; 41% of the deaths were due to cancer.(3) A similar outbreak, called Yu-Cheng, occurred in Taiwan in 1979. High concentrations of PCBs and also the more toxic polychlorinated dibenzofurans (PCDFs) (4) were present in the rice oil. The PCDGs were formed by heating the PCB in rice oil to 200 degrees C, at reduced pressure.(5) The outbreak caused 39 babies born from PCB-poisoned mothers to have hyperpigmentation and 24 of these died from either liver disfunction, liver cancer or infection. Numerous non-specific symptoms which persisted for years were reported in Yusho and Yu-Cheng patients.(6)

Some of the most common symptoms in Yusho and Yu-Cheng disease were:

- Disturbance of Vision
- Easy Fatigue
- Headache
- Reproductive impairment
- Malaise
- Numbness of limbs
- Pruritus
- Immune System Disfunction
- Dizziness
- Chloracne
- Eye discharge

Through the 1970's and 1980's many research projects have clearly shown the deadly results of PCB contamination. For example, in 1980, Kuratsune studied skin changes of chloracne, eye discharge and nail changes followed by infection and increased pigmentation. They discovered a dose-response relationship between skin changes and PCB levels.(3) Numerous other studies clearly demonstrated immune system disfunction, reproductive impairment, cancer, and hypertension complications. (7)(16)

Therefore, the proven existence of PCBs in all of our bodies is enough alone to create great concern knowing the damage this compound produces to our health. Yet, this is only one of the many thousands of toxins with damaging effects. Referring to the NHATS study discussed earlier, 100% of the U.S. population also carries in their bodies:

Styrene	- from styrene based disposable cups
	- Dichlorobenzene 1,4
	- from mothballs, house deodorizers
Xylene	- from gasoline, paints, and lacquers
Ethylphenol	- from drinking water
OCDD	- from wood treatment, herbicides, incinerators, auto exhausts

Also 90 to 100% of us carry the following toxic residues in our bodies:

1,2,3,4,6,7,8-**HpCDD**	- from wood treatment, herbicides, incinerators, auto exhausts
HxCDD	- from wood treatment, herbicides, incinerators, auto exhausts
Benzene	- from gasoline
Chlorobenzene	- from drinking water
Ethylbenzene	- from gasoline
p, p1-**DDE**	- from produce
1,2,3,4,6,7,7-**PeCDD**	- from wood treatment, herbicides, incinerators, auto exhausts
Toluene	- from gasoline

When one discovers the toxic damaging affects of these poisons, it should cause any serious minded person to become extremely nervous, even frightened. All of these toxic compounds have clearly documented destructive effects on our bodies. There are as yet many unknowns concerning just how serious this epidemic really is, yet there are enough knowns to clearly prove all of our bodies are being damaged internally in one way or another.

Let's take a little closer look at some specifics of how we are being poisoned. In 1988 the U.S. Department of the Interior released the following statement: "The national status of ground water contamination from toxic chemicals and organic substances cannot be quantified at present because of a lack of consistent data and basic knowledge of ground-water systems." Which means basically that the government can't figure out just how bad our water contamination really is! This report also continued, "All states also report some ground-water contamination from human activities such as landfills, fertilizers, pesticides, septic systems, underground storage tanks and chemicals spills." The report concluded by saying, "Available data. . .have led to a growing realization that toxic constituents and synthetic organic chemicals have contaminated shallow aquifers in many parts of the nation.

Reports of contamination are likely to increase as the search intensifies and more sophisticated techniques of detection are used." In 1991, over 9,000,000 wells were found to be contaminated with toxic chemicals.

Also in 1991, 350,000 toxic landfills or dumps were reported. Researchers have now discovered or identified over 700 chemicals in culinary drinking water! Yet the current national law, or standards by which local water systems are governed, states that, "Suppliers are required to monitor water supply periodically for 34 inorganic and organic contaminants." This law is known as the National Drinking Standards Act. With 700 possible chemicals identified in water and 34 tested for, does this give you the impression that our government has the ability to protect our population from contaminated water? It leaves me with no doubt that they cannot and do not have the technology or ability to provide safe drinking water.

Numerous pesticide residues are present in many foods. Many can linings contain phenolic resin, and many foods are treated with fumigants, fungicides, sulfur treatments, artificial colors, sweeteners, and preservatives. Ethylene is a gas used in ripening procedures, protective waxes, and packaging materials (plastics), all of which add to our toxic accumulation problems.

The current method to control pests and weeds for commercial produce growers are pesticides and herbicides. Scientists used to believe that micro amounts of chemicals both on and in our produce, placed there by farmers, were harmless to man. Their use therefore, has been approved by the agencies designed to protect food quality. However, there is now serious doubt and questions being raised by numerous scientists and researchers.

We have all heard about or know that the AIDS virus kills by attacking our immune system. This is an example of how important our immune function is to our health. As in AIDS, when our immune system becomes destroyed, we are left defenseless against all other invading microorganisms, which produce the secondary infections, that ultimately kill the AIDS victim. These body toxins, which we all have accumulating in our bodies, do the same type of thing, only slower and more subtly!

To substantiate that line of reasoning, let's take a look at the following quote from Frederick Kutz, one of our countries research biologists. He, representing the E.P.A., said: "For the first time there is clear and rather unequivocal evidence that the environmental exposure to pesticides at low levels causes cancer in man. It has taken a long time for that particular finding to emerge. The emergency of the new epidemiological data is cause for very serious concern. These toxic chemicals produce neurotixicity, immunotoxicity, and reproductive system damage."

An interesting study done in 1992 (Falck, F, et al: Pesticides and polychlorinated biphenyl residues in human breast lipids and their relation to breast cancer. Archives of Environmental health 47:143-6, 1992), evaluated the possible role to pesticides and pollutants in breast cancer. The levels of "Halogenated hydrocarbons" such as DDT, DDE, PCB, PCP, dieldrin, and chlordane, in fat cells of the breast were measured in women with malignant cancers in comparison to women with nonmalignant growth. Elevated levels of toxic pesticides were found in women with breast cancer compared to the women with benign breast disease. There appears to be a strong association between pesticide levels in breast tissue and breast cancer.

Most people don't realize that 1.2 billion pounds of pesticides and herbicides are sprayed or added to our crops each year. Experts estimate that only 2% of the pesticide actually serves its purpose while over 98% of the pesticide is absorbed into the air, water, soil, or food supply. In 1984, the National Resource Defense Council conducted a survey of fresh produce sold in San Francisco markets for pesticide residues and found 44% of 71 fruit and vegetables had detectable levels of 19 different pesticides with 42% of the produce with detectable pesticide residues containing more than one pesticides, (Mott L and Broad M: Pesticides in Food. National Resources Defense Council. San Francisco, CA 1984). Over 50 different pesticides are used on broccoli, 110 on apples, 70 on bell peppers according to (Quillin P: Safe Eating. Evans, New York, NY, 1990).

I assume that you now realize that most of the fruits, vegetables, and grains which you and your families have been eating for years have been contaminated with micro amounts of pesticides and herbicides. If you now suffer from Multiple Chemical Sensitivity, you will be more fascinated with the materials contained in this first chapter. I feel it is necessary to provide you with a reasonable background into the cause of this bio-accumulation epidemic.

A federal committee formed 20 years ago to study the effects of pesticides came up with an interesting conclusion and statement when they said, "Pesticide toxicology exemplifies the absurdity of the situation in which 200 million Americans are undergoing lifelong exposure, yet our knowledge of what is happening to them is fragmentary."

More than 50,000 pesticides are in use today. Americans have used pesticides on crops, yards, homes, schools and work places for more than 40 years. Most Americans for decades have eaten minuscule amounts, low levels as Frederick Kutz calls them, of many pesticides in their fruits, vegetables, grains, and other foods. These various toxin sources result in a cumulative effect on the whole body when they combine with other chemicals in meat, poultry, air and water!

The world health organization has reported that 20,000 people a year have died in the past 4 years, worldwide, from pesticide exposure.

Federally permissible traces of various pesticides and drugs exist in much of the meat and poultry that Americans consume. The Federal Government actually inspects less than 1% of the meat consumed in the U.S. every year. And when it is inspected, it is done so by methods used to detect only a few potential chemical contaminants.

The following true story demonstrates a drastic chain of events ending in human contamination. In the early 1970's, the toxic fire retardant PBB was accidentally substituted for a nutritional supplement for farm animals. The resulting contamination of meat, milk and a number of other foods ended with the ingestion of the chemical by virtually the entire population of Michigan. Victims of this disaster had been the subjects of intensive study by a clinical research team from Mount Sinai School of Medicine who found that 97% of the 1000 state residents had PBB 0.2 ppb or more by 1978. There was clear evidence of widespread health effects. (Wolff et al.JAMA 1982 PBB.) They also concluded that there had been no significant reduction of PBB levels over the six year period following the contamination. Their conclusion was that the PBB was there to stay.

Our meat and poultry have not yet reached these levels, still it is contaminated, and it is definitely effecting us!

People eat a lot of fish or seafoods. In fact in 1988, Americans ate fish or shellfish once a week for an annual total of 15.4 pounds for every person, according to the National Fisheries Institute. Also in 1988, a non-profit, Washington-based group, called the Center for Science in the Public Interest, issued this gloomy conclusion, "To one degree or another, fish from any body of water are potential repositories of industrial chemicals, pesticides or toxic metals." The scope of health problems from contaminated seafood alone, is potentially enormous!!

Many, if not most, of our nation's coastal waters and streams have become open sewers teaming with chemicals, poisons and human waste. Many Americans, attempting to reduce cholesterol, are turning from red meats to fish and seafood as an alternative. Yet the presence of toxic bio-accumulations in fish, is perhaps worse than the cholesterol threat. At a time when our streams and oceans are badly contaminated with chemicals and waste, fish and seafood still remain the only flesh foods not required to be federally inspected.

Polynuclear aromatic hydrocarbons, P.H.A.'s which are created by a variety of urban-pollution sources, now circulate in most urban air basins at levels high enough to cause genetic mutations in the livers of laboratory rats. Although rats are not people, you can be assured that this pollution is not helping our livers either!! CO, (carbon monoxide) mostly from auto exhaust, is also a common offender with a hemoglobin affinity of 245 times that of O_2 to function. Research indicates a much higher incidence of athero-sclerosis due to high CO levels.

Many people are somewhat aware of the facts concerning outdoor air quality, mainly because it can be seen! And it is true that outdoor air quality is something that we all need to be very concerned with, and do something about!! However, I would like the reader to know that a much worse problem with air quality exists. According to [Nero, A., "Controlling Indoor Air Pollution," Scientific American (1988) 258(5):42-48] the average person sustains much greater exposures indoors than out, usually 20:1 greater exposure. (20 times worse indoor air pollution.) There are two basic methods for creating a bio-accumulation problem from indoor air.

1.   A massive, overwhelming exposure @ chemical spill, fire with synthetic material, pesticide spraying, working with chemicals in a confined, unventilated space.
2.   Or, for most of us, repeated, low-level exposure to a complex array of synthetic organic compounds @ diesel exhaust, tight buildings, etc.

Some of the many offenders for polluting indoor air quality are: gas stoves, gas or oil-fired furnaces and space heaters, central air heating, sponge rubber bedding padding, and upholstery, various plastics, such as shower curtains, insecticides, perfumes, paint and decorating materials, fireplaces, cleaning agents, disinfectants, deodorizers, mothballs, cedar closets, newsprint, various fabrics, particleboard, carpeting and padding, disinfectant liquids and sprays containing phenolics. (Miksch R.R., Hollowell, C.D., Schmidt, H.E. "Trace Organic Chemical Contaminants in Office Space," Environ Int. 8:129-138, 1982).

To illustrate this point and the severity and potential

danger of indoor air quality, I would like to relate the following tragic but true stories.

In 1985, the Iglesias family purchased a 32 acre farm in Kaufman County, Texas. They were buying their dream, a place where they could raise their only child and live the kind of simple, clean life that they had worked so hard for.

The farm was then treated for termites with chlordane by Environmental Pest Control Systems (EPCS), a privately owned exterminator company.

A few months later, when the Iglesias family moved in, the farm was plagued with scorpions. The Iglesias' feared for their child's safety so they asked EPCS to help them with the scorpion problem. Little did they know that EPCS had not only misapplied the initial application of chlordane, but they would misapply three consecutive sprayings for scorpions! Years later the Igesias' would finally realize that EPCS had misapplied the pesticide, violated FIFRA (Federal Insecticide, Fungicide, and Rodenticide Act) regulations, and operated without insurance. However, the process of realizing the EPCS had indeed harmed their family and broke the law was a slow and painful one for them to understand.

The entire family began experiencing illnesses almost immediately upon moving into their new home. They first attributed the illnesses to the flu, allergies, or other problems. Doctors told them they had viruses and treated them with antibiotics: however the flu didn't go away, the allergies showed no relief, and the logical explanations were no longer logical. Daisy, their daughter, tested negative for allergies and Cystic Fibrosis, but she continued to have chronic, sever vomiting and diarrhea, itching and rashes, leg and stomach pains, balance problems, and unexplained heavy salivating. In addition, she began to develop personality changes.

Elizabeth and Luis experienced similar symptoms in addition to headaches, heart palpitation, eye problems, muscles jerking, facial tics, night sweats, depression, and chronic fatigue. Luis experienced extreme testicular pain, and Elizabeth began to have unusual menstrual problems. Their personality changes took the form of unexplained rages, deep depression, erratic or lethargic behavior and Elizabeth thought she was going crazy.

As time went on Daisy began showing more alarming symptoms. Blood tests revealed that there was 2 1/2 times the exposed adult level of pesticide metabolites in her blood. Her blood tests also revealed an indication of leukemia, bone marrow cancer and liver abnormalities. Luis developed tumors and eventually sarcoma cancer; Elizabeth developed 15 separate tumors.

The Iglesias' animals started to get sick. A veterinarian diagnosed their horse as dying of lymphosarcoma cancer and six months later two family dogs died of sarcoma cancer.

Elizabeth began to suspect that the pesticide applications were responsible for their illnesses and her animals' deaths. She began to investigate what happened and what these chemical could do. Elizabeth found that her baby had been exposed to Chlordane, Heptachlor, Chlorpynfus and Diazinon. She also found that the first application of chlordane was misapplied in the crawl space of the house. This set the stage for the initial exposure and the onset of their health problems. Then the applicator sprayed three more times with chlordane and other chemicals to kill scorpions. (At that time FIFRA regulations authorized that chlordane could only be used on subsurface application of termite control.) This was just one of many direct FIFRA violations. He then continued to spray around the outside exposing the animals directly and local winds carried the chemical to the pastures. These chemicals were found in the air, on Daisy's toys, in the carpet, four feet above the baseboard on the wall and in the closets. The Iglesias' had to leave their home and all their life long possessions. Today, the farm remains lifeless and deadly.

In the preceding six years, the Iglesias' have had to face homelessness, a splitting up of a family, total financial ruin, and failure of the medical and legal systems. Their illnesses have worsened and they have not received any compensation. The world they knew in 1986 is gone forever and Elizabeth fights every day for the health of her daughter and the protection of other victimized families across this nation. She has vowed never to allow this to happen to another family. "My daughter's future is uncertain. I am not so much interested in compensation to get money except to help my daughter, but I am wanting justice for all the loss and suffering my family has endured. My story is only one of thousands. It doesn't make me feel good that I am not alone in this dilemma."

Final Note - the applicator sold his company immediately after he was reported to authorities. Many other families are claiming misapplications and to date he has never been adequately investigated!!

The reader may ask themselves, "Do I really know what is being done to my home when pest control companies do their thing?" Our homes should be a safe haven of love and peace, not a place of contamination, a death trap!

There are several basic suggestions for making our homes a safer environment such as eliminating ventless combustion appliances, carefully selecting stable building and furnishing materials, preventing the exposure of unstable materials to heat and sunlight, and the careful choice and use of electric appliances.

The EPA did a study in 1987 on over 400 residents in New Jersey, North Carolina and North Dakota. They were looking at 40 different V.O.C.'s, (volatile organic compounds) CO, (carbon monoxide) pesticides, particulates, and comparing indoor and outdoor toxic levels, measuring individual exposures and resulting body burdens and carcinogenic organic chemicals. They found that everyone of the 40 VOC's studied had higher indoor levels than outdoor. These higher indoor levels or VOC's were being emitted from numerous materials, including: building materials, furnishings, dry-cleaned clothes, gasoline, hot showers, painted materials, etc. (EPA "the TEAM study" - total exposure assessment methodology. Wallace, L. et al., 1987.) A 1990 Immerman study also found indoor air quality dramatically worse than outdoor air quality particularly associated with various pesticides.

One more associated true, but tragic story may help to drive my warnings of the bioaccumulation threat deep into your conscious.

Over the last 16 years, the Boyds have endured blatant discrimination, contamination of their home, health and financial ruin, lies, cover ups and manipulation of the truth by a "nationally known company," the state and federal governments and others who were involved with their poisoning.

In July of 1977, Mr. and Mrs. Boyd and their five healthy children moved into a wonderful home. The home had been treated for termites by the original owner and showed no signs of termite infestation when the Boyds bought it and moved in.

Sometime in August of 1977, this company came to the Boyd's house and misrepresented nonexistent problems. The Boyd's claim that the solicitor told them they "might" have termites in places that can't be seen, and that the house could be "eaten down" and destroyed in a short period of time. According to the Boyds it was further claimed that because they lived near a creek they would have more insects. The solicitor convinced the Boyds they needed a "preventive contract." The solicitor based his remarks on NOT knowledge, but slick sales pitches designed to sell an unnecessary service. (It is important to know that during this time EPA prohibited manufactures from making chlordane because of suspected health problems but still gave applicators the right to use all remaining stock.)

During the company's initial treatment of the Boyd's home they illegally removed previous chemical barriers. Holes were drilled inside and outside to the foundation walls six to twelve inches apart and, in some places, there were two holes right on top of each other. The holes were too high according to application standards and were applied in improper void areas. They drilled holes next to ventilation systems and in the kitchen areas. All of the holes were left uncovered. This was all done with no signs of termite infestation!

In February 1978, the Georgia Department of Agriculture (GDA), came to the Boyd's home claiming to be doing a "routine inspection" on the company. They visually inspected the house and announced to the Boyds that they were going to make the company come back and retreat the house. Between May and June of 1978 the company retreated the Boyd's home under direct order from the State. Still there was no proof that there were termites on the property. During this time the applicator spilled chemicals in the carport and the yard. The children walked through the spilled chemicals resulting in direct contact to their skin. Shortly thereafter, the skin on their legs and feet peeled off. Again the same holes were saturated with chemicals and left uncovered. The GDA was not at the second spraying to supervise the company.

The Boyd's health problems began after the first treatment and worsened after each treatment. Their symptoms included headaches, confusion, irritability, muscle weakness, vision problems, upset stomach, vomiting, cramps, dizziness, disorientation, bowel irritation, skin rashes and eruptions. Each time the furnace was turned on, the odors would fill the house and they would all get sick. They lived in a constant state of ill health, mounting doctor bills and fear of the unknown.

As part of the preventive contract, the company began to spray the Boyd's home on a monthly basis with various toxic chemicals. Mr. Boyd expressed his concern regarding the repeated treatments and the effects on his family, but the applicator argued with him and accused him of questioning his authority and job performance. He guaranteed the Boyds that these chemicals would not harm them and that residual odors would be gone within 48 hours. The Boyd family became extremely ill so Mr. Boyd demanded that the company not return. The applicator then accused the Boyds of trying to get out of the contract. In good faith Mr. Boyd paid for the remaining contract and kept them from any further spraying. By this time, the Boyds had four major treatments to their home in less than three years and had been sprayed on a monthly basis for several months. The Boyds later learned that their property had been contaminated with Chlordane, chlorohepton, malathion, pyrethrum, Diazinon granules, Dursban, R.D. 98 (a diazinon-pyrethrin dust formulation) and Copper Napthaenate, a fungus control. This does not name the inert ingredients mixed with the insecticides nor the combinations of insecticides mixed at the time of application.

The seven members of the Boyd family were now living in their kitchen. Because of the furnace distributing the contamination throughout the house, they had to block off all of the vents, turn off the heat in the dead of winter and close off the rest of the rooms.

Believe it or not, the worse is yet to come! The Lab, when doing the testing, withheld testing results from the Boyds and there was evidence that the results were not reported correctly. Later the Boyds found out that the lab contracted from the State and the applicator. The State continued to tell the Boyds that there was nothing wrong and covered up their part in the treatment process. The federal government continued to negate the severity of their problems: and finally, an unprepared lawyer allowed the Boyds to go to court where Mr. and Mrs. Boyd were demeaned and humiliated by being accused of poisoning their own family for monetary gain.

The children's symptoms advanced to paralysis, night sweats and terrors, and the inability to function in a normal manner. Mr. Boyd suffered respiratory failure on several occasions while Mrs. Boyd had neurological disorders. Eventually Mr. Boyd was injured on the job and was unable to work. It is suspected that his injury could have been a direct result of his exposure. They did not know what to do or where to turn.

An independent contractor hired by the Boyds, conducted a thorough inspection of their home and found extremely high levels of chlordane. The inspector found contamination in floors, and all surface layers, in the furniture, curtains, walls, baseboards, vents and crawl spaces. The house was poisoned! The Boyds were forced to leave all life long possessions and memories behind. The house still stands as a reminder of the violence that was brought against them.

Today the Boyds are hanging on by a thread. They are all still having severe health problems. The medical bills are still overwhelming resulting in severe financial problems. The VA (Veterans Administration) still threatens to foreclose on the house even though it has been condemned. The Boyds have had to declare bankruptcy. They live with the knowledge that any one of them at any time could have respiratory failure, contract a deadly disease or die from their exposure-related health problems. Their older children have given up their dreams to go to college because all of the savings and current income goes to supporting the family day by day.

The Boyd's two youngest children need medical testing to substantiate their claims of permanent damage and to open up the possibility of litigation for proper medical care. Mr. Boyd is aware it is too late to help himself, his wife, or his older children, but his dream is to help his two younger children and to continue to tell his story so that others won't experience the family devastation that they did.

Most people hope that some governmental agency or licensing division will control or regulate this type of problem. The problem is that most of the people in charge, are not aware of this problem. Many of the preceding mistakes were done in ignorance. If this book does nothing else but to make the reader more aware of the the environmental threat, and protect yourselves, it will have accomplished a majority of its' purpose.

The information and materials being presented here are not theoretical or someone's opinion. These are cold hard facts! Noted scientists from around the world concur that these toxins are slowly deteriorating our health, and if left unchecked, will ultimately lead to our ill health or early demise.

A few years ago, Dr. Joe Weissman, assistant clinical

professor of medicine at U.C.L.A. medical school, said; "Most physicians are taught that cancer rates have not changed much over time. But today, 1 in 4 or 25% of the population will come down with cancer. Soon, that figure will be one out of three people!"

I strongly believe that one of the primary reasons for increased cancers, immune disorders, and reproductive disorders, is toxic accumulations of body burdens, or toxic bio-accumulations.

Donald Kennedy, when head of the F.D.A., stated the environmental pollution threat this way, "Reasonable estimates are that not more than 5% of human cancer is due to viruses and less than 5% is due to radiation. Some 90% of cancer in man is, therefore, due to the chemicals."!!!

According to the U.S. Internal Trade Commission, synthetic organic chemical production in the U.S. from 1945 to 1985 indicated that levels are dramatically increasing.

1945 - approximately 9 million tons were produced.
1950 - approximately 11 million tons were produced.
1955 - approximately 16 million tons were produced.
1960 - approximately 23 million tons were produced.
1965 - approximately 41 million tons were produced.
1970 - approximately 63 million tons were produced.
1975 - approximately 75 million tons were produced.
1980 - approximately 110 million tons were produced.
1985 - approximately 112 million tons were produced.

All of these toxins also greatly promote the rapid formation or production of free radical oxygen molecules. These in turn wreak havoc in our bodies.

Dr. Elmer Cranton, M.D., one of our country's leading chelation doctors, and Arline Brecher wrote a book titled "Bypassing Bypass," where in part they described the damaging effects of Free Radicals in our bodies. Some of the following are quotes from that book.

Our bodies are composed of about 60 trillion cells, each enclosed within an encircling cell wall of membrane. Cells are continuously worn out and have the ability to replace themselves. Other tissues, such as the brain, nerves and muscles (including the heart) are made up of non-dividing cells that, once worn out, cannot renew themselves. Over time, nonrenewable cells become increasingly damaged in the course of their activities: they age, they die, and they clog tissues and organs and biochemical pathways as cellular "rubbish." When your cells are damaged, you are damaged. When your cells perform inefficiently, you perform inefficiently.

Free radical is an oxygen molecule with an odd number of electrons in the orbital ring of one of its' atoms. Free radicals differ from all other molecules, ions, and molecular complexes in having an unpaired electron in their structure.

If one of the electrons in a pair becomes separated, an imbalance is created. That imbalance makes the resulting molecule (or atom) promiscuously unstable, violently reactive, and very destructive, ready to aggressively attack any nearby substance, setting off further free radical reactions with explosive cell-destroying power.

What the free radicals actually do is combine with and react chemically with other molecules that were never meant to be interfered with, just as outside of us oxygen produces rust on metal surfaces, so inside of us, unbalanced oxygen molecules "rust" the body.

Uncontrolled, these free radicals can cause extreme damage to the body. They are deadly marauders that damage cells by breaking down delicate cell walls, by damaging important protein enzymes, and by ravaging the sensitive structures of the Mitochondria so that it is no longer an efficient energy producer. Free radicals have a live-span of micro-seconds and their concentration in any site any moment is minuscule, but they will attack anything in their vicinity with amazing speed.

There is absolutely no way to escape ongoing exposure. Even before the nuclear age, man was constantly subjected to radiation. One quart of ordinary air on a sunny day contains about 1 billion free radicals of a highly dangerous form of ozone. Radiation from the sun and stars continually filters through the atmosphere subjecting our bodies to free radical exposure.

In a healthy body, free radical reactions are controlled by still being allowed to proceed in an orderly fashion as needed for energy production and for detoxification of chemicals, germs, and foreign substances. Several enzymes (including Catalase, Superoxide Dismutase, and Glutathione Peroxdase in cooperation with other anti-oxidants) keep free radicals from running wild. When functioning properly, these enzymes, in concert with an elaborate system of natural free radical scavengers (including the antioxidant vitamins, C and E and pycnogenol) dampen free radical chemical reactions, thus allowing the desired biological effect without unwanted cellular or molecular damage.

The damage is cumulative and progressive. If the rate of free radical production proceeds unchecked, eventually the body's natural defenses are overwhelmed. Once the containment threshold is breached, concentration of free radicals is increased by a million fold.

The resulting cell destruction, malignant mutation, and damage to enzymes lead to the whole spectrum of circulatory, malignant, inflammatory, and immunologic disorders that cause the vast majority of age-related illness.

Our biological time clock, which begins ticking at birth, seems to run at a speed determined by our bodys' efficiency in taking command of free radical chemical reactions.

Reduced defenses against destructive free radical activity accelerates, the aging process.

Virtually everyone is internally contaminated. Your good health is being attacked. A study by Ashford et al. 1984, suggested that the underlying cause of interindividual variability, (why some people get sick or experience more symptoms than others) include age, sex, genetic makeup, lifestyle and behavioral factors such as nutritional factors and dietary factors: alcohol, tobacco, drug use, etc. Various environmental factors and preexisting diseases also play a role. However, it doesn't matter if you are feeling symptoms or not, the inescapable and frightening fact remains that your body is contaminated with toxic residues from our environment. These toxins do rapidly produce free radical oxygen molecules. Everyone is effected to one degree or another because their environment is sick!!. Your condition may be subclinical (not detectable by clinical tests), or a premorbid state (before the detectable disease begins), or asymptomatic (not causing any symptoms).

My purpose here is not to frighten or cause panic, but to educate, and hopefully cause you to take action. We all need to take personal responsibility to create the needed change.

Some of the common, often recurring, symptoms associated with toxic bio-accumulations include: headaches, fatigue, mental confusion, lack of mental acuity, memory loss, flu like symptoms, irritability, eye and mucous membrane irritations, skin disorders, musculoskeletal pains, and increased irritations to dust and pollens. Other possible health effects which may be associated with toxic accumulations and a condition known as Multiple Chemical Sensitivity include: obesity, cardiovascular disease, EENT disorders, endocrine disorders, gastrointestinal disorders, hematological abnormalities, neurobehavioral and psychiatric manifestations, neurological disorders, pulmonary disorders, renal and urological disorders, rheumatological disorders.

However, if you do not have any of these symptoms, it doesn't mean that you are not effected! You are!! Research proves this! Often symptoms are simply your bodys' way of finally telling you that it can't take much more!!

Americans have, what scientists call, one of the lowest health indexes of any industrial society on the planet. One of the main reasons for this, is that most of us have the false idea that the time to do something, (to seek health care), is after we have the illness, disease, cancer or whatever. We simply do not truly understand the concepts of prevention very well. The vast majority of health care providers would readily agree that healthy living principles applied consistently, daily, will prevent many or most illnesses.

The following are a few more facts relating to bioaccumulations:

According to the U.S. EPA, by 1980 over 400 chemicals had been identified in human tissues, with some 48 found in adipose tissue, 40 in milk, 73 in liver tissues and over 250 in blood.

The predominant storage compartment within the human body is the fat. We therefore look to toxins which have been found within this tissue as some of the main offenders.

Dr. Nicholas Ashford wrote in "The New England Journal of Medicine," and called for health scientists to begin formulating policies for preventing chemically induced illness rather than waiting for "bodies to fall."

The "Journal of the American Medical Association" reported in 1986 that Kansas farmers exposed to herbicides more than 20 days each year were far more likely to contract Non-Hodgkins lymphoma than those who weren't exposed.

Dr. David Prescott and Abraham Flexer in a 1982 book entitled "Cancer, the Misguided Cell" amplified Kennedy's thoughts this way: "These carcinogens, particularly chemicals of various kinds, are in the foods we eat, in the air we breath, in the water we drink and the clothes we wear . . . the amounts and variety . . . have increased sharply in the last 25 years . . . and they continue to increase rapidly."

Interaction of toxic chemicals with critical DNA-rearranging enzyme proteins causes malfunction in immune reactive cells. (18) This type of interaction can cause cell death or the generation of an oncogene, (tumor forming gene), which in turn develops into an inheritable mutation and gradually into a malignancy.

Toxic bio-accumulations are also suspect in the triggering of a previously quiescent oncogene (previously dormant), and the gradual development of a malignancy. (19)

Reference list for chapter one:

1. U.S. Environmental Protection Agency, " Broad Scan Analysis of the FY82 National Human Adipose Tissue Survey Specimens", EPA-560/5-86-035, December, 1986.

2. Wolff, M.S., Anderson, H.A., Selikoff, I.J., Human Tissue Burdens of Aromatic Chemicals in Michigan, J.A.M.A. 247: 2112-2116, 1982.

3. Kuratsune, M., Yusho, In: Halogenated Biophenyls, Terphenyls, Naphthalenes, Dibenzodioxins and Related Products. Ed. Kimbrough, R.D., Elsevier/North-Holland Biomedical Pres, Amsterdam, pp. 373-397, 1980.

4. Kunita, N., et al., Biological effects of PCBs, PCQs and PCDFs in the Oil Causing Yusho and Yu-Cheng, Environ. Health Persp. 59: 79-84, 1985.

5. Masuda, Y., et al., PCB and PCKF Congeners in the Blood and Tissue of Yusho and Yu-Cheng Patients, Environ. Health Persp. 59: 53-58, 1985.

6. Landrigan, P.J., General Population Exposure to Environmental Concentrations of Halogenated

Biphenyls, In: Halogenated Biphenyls, Terphenyls, Haphthalenes, Dibenzodioxins and Related Products, Ed. Kimbrough, R.D., Elsevier/North-Holland Biomedical Pres, Amsterdam, pp 373-397, 1980.

7. Vos, J.G. and Van Driel Grootenhuis, L., PCB Induced Suppression of the Humoral and Cell - Mediated Immunity in Guinea Pigs. Sci Total Environ. 1:289-302, 1972.

8. Lee, T.P., Chang, K.J., Health Effects of PCBs, In: Immunotoxicology and Immunopharmacology, Ed Dean, J.H., Raven Press, New York, pp. 415-422, 1985.

9. Yamashitu, F. and Hayashi, M., Fetal PCB Syndrome: Clinical Features, Intrauterine Growth Retardation and Possible Alteration in Calcium Metabolism, Environ. Health Persp. 59:41-45, 1985.

10. Barsotti, D.A., Marlar, R.J. and Allen, J.R. Reproductive Dysfunction in Rhesus Monkeys Exposed to Low Levels of Polychlorinated Biphenyls (Aroclor 1248), Fd. Cosmet. Toxicol. 14:99-103, 1976.

11. Togan, W.J., Neonatal Effects to Transplacental Exposure to PCBs and DDE, J. Pediatrics 109:336-341, 1986.

12. National Cancer Institute, Bioassay of Aroclor 1254 for Possible Carcinogenicity, CAS #27323-18-8, NTIS Springfield, VA PB-279 624/1 GA NCI-CG TR-38. DHEW/Pub. NCI, Washington, D.C. 1977, NIH78-838.

13. Bertazzi, P.a. et al., Cancer Mortality of Capacitor Manufacturing Workers, Am. J. Ind. Med. 11:257-264, 1987.

14. Kreiss, K., et al., Association of Blood Pressure and poly-chlorinated Biphenyl levels, J.A.M.A. 245:2505-2509, 1981.

15. Pines, A., et al., Levels of Some Organochlorine Residues in Blood Patients with Arteriosclerotic

Disease, Sci. Total Environ. 54:135-155, 1986.

16. Akaji, K. and Okumura, M., Association of Blood Pressure and PCB Level in Yusho Patients, Environ. Health Persp. 59:37-39, 1985.

17. Safe, S., Metabolism, Uptake, Storage and Bioaccumulation, In: Halogenated Biphenyls, Terphenyls, Haphthalenes, Dibenzodioxins and Related Products, Ed. Kimbrough, R.D., Elsevier/North-Holland Biomedical Press, Amsterdam, pp. 373-379, 1980.

18. Shuurman, H.(1991). Chemicals trophic for thymus and T cells: Risk for immunodeficiency and autoimmunity. Proceedings of 5th International Congress on Immunopharmacy. May 26-31.

19. Levin A.S., Multiple Chemical Sensitivities: A practicing Clinician's Point of View Clinical and Immunologic Research Findings. Toxicology & Industrial Health, Vol. 8, Number 4, 1992.

Chapter Two

THE DEVELOPMENT OF THE CHIROHOLISTIC DETOXIFICATION TREATMENT PROGRAM

Studying this information, and realizing the negative implications to our health, I eagerly set out to do something about it as a doctor. It was in the Fall of 1986, when I began to employ some of the discoveries I had been making about methods of reducing some of these toxic body burdens. This was the beginning of what is now known as the "Chiroholistic Detoxification Treatment Program." I first learned that if people would drink large quantities of pure water daily it would assist in flushing toxic residues from the body through various cleansing systems such as the urinary tract and intestinal tract. At this time I also began prescribing what I called detox baths, which were treatments designed to elevate body core temperature and elicit perspiration response, which also provided another route for the elimination of these toxic residues.

I should point out that heat treatments should be used with caution and best under a doctors supervision with this application. Hyperthermia, a condition of excessive heat build up in the body, causes various physiologic reactions, some potentially dangerous, and need to be guarded against. Heat treatments also are ill advised for hypertensive individuals, individuals with certain nerve pathologies or patients with certain circulatory disorders. Also because heat treatments have a lipophilic toxin mobilizing effect, (1) other reactions can occur, which a trained doctor would know how to deal with effectively.

In this early stage of the detoxification program I also utilized various nutritional supplements to help prevent dehydration and promote toxin mobilization. I also encouraged limited sunbathing in our early program.

From the beginning of the program, I attempted to speed up the movement through the intestinal tract. Therefore, I always recommended increasing the intake of all kinds of palatable vegetables, fruits, grains, seeds, etc. With the increased fiber, and retention of water, the result would be a faster moving bowel. I worked with the patients until they achieved 2 or 3 B.M's. per day.

I continued with this early form of the detox program until 1987-88. When I began using these various methods, I was pleased with the results. I had great success with some of the stubborn cases I previously had not been able to help. The patients who couldn't find help elsewhere, were happy with the results we were getting.

Then in mid 1988, a new patient by the name of Robert came to my office and wanted to go through my detoxification program. After I told him of the various methods I was using, he explained that he had just completed a treatment program at Health Med in California. He told me that his treatment at Health Med was very similar to the one that I was doing. This was most interesting to me because until this point, I wasn't familiar with any other available treatment methods for this problem. Robert was kind enough to share with me all of his information from Health Med, which I was intrigued with. This information had reference to many different research projects which were dealing with bio-accumulation, environmental illness and multiple chemical sensitivity. I immediately contacted the various research groups and obtained copies of the research materials for myself. In studying this vast array of research materials, I was introduced to various groups and organizations involved in helping people suffering with bio-accumulation.

After digesting this new information, I discovered several new and greatly needed techniques to help my detox program. I discovered that certain types of physical exercise had a mobilizing effect on lipophilic toxins. (2) I discovered that several other detoxification programs utilized jogging for 20 to 30 minutes followed by a sauna. Yet I knew that jogging would exclude many potential patients who suffered from this ailment. I had also been previously studying the therapeutic effects of rebounding, or jumping on a mini-trampoline. This exercise not only would mobilize toxins but probably do it much more efficiently due to the positive, negative "G" forces at work. This action also had some very therapeutic effects on the lymphatic circulation. Therefore, because of this knowledge, and many other benefits of rebounding, I chose this method of mobilizing toxins instead of jogging.

I also took a hard look at the type of heat treatment I wanted to employ in my program. The sauna was effective, however I believed the detox bath is superior. The ideal detox bath should be in purified water to prevent absorption of chemicals from the contaminated water. A water bath provided a greatly superior skin surface contact in heating the body core over moist sauna air. The liquid medium was able to transfer heat more readily, and various therapeutic substances could also be added to the water to even promote detoxification faster. I found it necessary to be very careful in administering heat treatments as I discussed earlier. Temperatures could be easily modified for different individual needs. However, 102 to 105 F seemed to be the ideal in most cases. Most patients are advised to completely submerge to their ears for 20 min. Certain preliminary skin treatment is recommended prior to entrance into the detox bath.

Upon further evaluation of the available researched materials on this subject, I found that there has been quite a number of research projects which specifically looked at the effectiveness of this type of detoxification program. (1)(3)(5)(6)

Several doctors in the U.S. have been utilizing detoxification methods similar to the methods originally developed for Health Med. Before and after lab studies demonstrate an impressive decrease in various bio-accumulates such as DDT, PCB's, DDE, PBB, HCB, DIELDRIN, etc. These toxins generally are reduced from 30 to 97%. And most patients experience a great decrease in toxin associated symptoms.

As learned in chapter 1, any effective clinical detoxification program must also effectively deal with, and include an effective antioxidant therapy. Or an effective method of scavenging and neutralizing the free radical toxic oxygen created from numerous sources.

Some of these sources besides accumulating toxic pesticides and toxic herbicides include:
- radiation from sunlight and x-ray,
- trapped ozone in the atmosphere,
- cured meats, asbestos, carcinogens of all sorts,
- phenobarbital, chemotherapy, air pollution,
- excessive exercise, heat, tobacco smoke, physical trauma, infection, stress, and alcohol.

You may also be interested that free radical production alone has been linked or implicated in more than sixty diseases, including among other: Alzheimer's, Parkinson's, AIDS, cancer, arthritis, rheumatism, cataracts, kidney disorders, liver disorders, heart attack, stroke, sickle cell anemia, senility, edema, phlebitis, swollen extremities, cold toes, cold fingers, and strangely enough jet lag.

For example: Parkinson's is a brain condition that produces muscle tremor, stiffness, and weakness. The usual symptoms include trembling rigid posture, slow movements, and a shuffling and unbalanced gate. The exact cause of Parkinson's is still a mystery, however it is believed that neurotoxins cause oxidative damage to the basal ganglia in the brain tissues. And it is the responsibility of the basal ganglia to control muscle tension and movement. In the oxidative model, oxidation reactions lead to the generation of free radicals - which are capable of destroying the cell membranes and nerve cells.

It is most interesting to note that in a study (Fabn S: A pilot trial of high0dose alpha-tocopherol and ascorbate in early Parkinson's disease. Annals of Neurology 32:S128-32, 1992), antioxidants have been shown to slow the progress of Parkinson's. In 1979, Vitamins C and E were administered to 21 patients with early Parkinson's disease were given 3,000 mg of vitamin C and 3,200 IU of vitamin E each day. The patients were followed closely for a period of seven years. Although all patients eventually required drug treatment (Sinemet of Deprenyl), the progression of the disease as determined by need for medication was considerably delayed in those receiving the nutritional antioxidants, for up to 2 to 3 years longer. these results are very promising for Parkinson's patients particularly since Pycnogenol readily bypasses the blood brain barrier and is much more powerful than the antioxidants C and E.

Since 1981, I knew that a number of vitamins, bioflavonoids, and minerals had reported antioxidant properties. Some of the most common are vitamins E and C and beta-carotene. However all of these had limited bio-availability (limited absorption into the blood stream and cellular uptake), and were short lived in the body, lasting only two to four hours. Also some of the commonly bioflavonoids were toxic, taken in higher dosage or prolonged periods of time. So I began looking for something that was better.

I came across an interesting story, re-told by Dr. Masquelier who eventually discovered what I as looking for.

Since this story, is worth repeating, I will in a condensed version:

"In 1534 French explorer Jacques Cartier was blocked by ice in the Gulf of St. Lawrence. His crew was forced to subsist on their rations of salted meat and biscuits. Eventually, this diet, which was completely void of vegetables and fruits, led to the onset of scurvy. Soon twenty-five of his 110-man crew had died, and more than 50 others were seriously ill."

"Since Mid-November until April 15, we were continuously trapped by five feet of ice and four feet of snow such that it was higher than the decks of our ships. The entire river was frozen above Hochelaga. Thus it was that we lost 25 of our best men to the dreaded sickness. There were another forty who were at the point of death and the remainder, except two or three, were all gravely ill. But God, in his infinite grace, took pity on us and provided us with the knowledge and the remedy for our cure and health in the manner set forth below.

How, by the grace of God, we came to know about a certain tree by which were cured: and all the sick recovered after having used it: and the manner of its use.

One day, our captain, taking note of the spreading sickness, and the condition of his men, left the fort and, walking on the ice, observed a group of people from Stadacone, among whom was Agaya, whom the captain had seen ten or twelve days before suffering from the same illness that affected our crew; one of his legs had shrunk to the size of a two year old's at the knee with all loss of sensation, he had lost most of his teeth and the remaining teeth were rotten along with rotted and infected gums. The captain, seeing Agaya healthy and alert was overjoyed, hoping to learn of the circumstances of the cure, and how he might help his own crew. When they arrived at the fort, the captain questioned him concerning his cure. Agaya responded that he was cured with the liquid and residue from the leaves of a tree, and that was the sole cure for the illness. The captain asked him if there were any such trees in the vicinity of the fort and told him that his cabinboy had come down with an illness, not wishing to let Agaya know the extent to which his crew had been affected.

At that point Agaya sent two women with our captain and they gathered nine or ten branches; and they showed us how to strip the leaves and pull the bark from the branches, and to boil them in water, then to drink the water every other day, and to put the drugs on the inflamed legs. They informed him that the tree cured all maladies. In their language, the tree is called annedda.

Shortly thereafter, the captain made a beverage for the sick members of the crew of whom only one or two were courageous enough to try it. As soon as they had taken it, they asked for more which turned out to be a miracle as for every illness with which they were afflicted, they were cured and restored to health after having drunk the brew only two or three times: such that the crew who had syphilis for five or six years were completely cured.

After having seen all that, the crew was ready to kill to get the medicine. This wonderful tree has done in less than a week what all the physicians of Louvain and Montpelier, using all the drugs of Alexandria, would not be able to accomplish in a year. Thanks to God, everyone who used the remedy was cured and restored to good health."

Four centuries later, Jack Masquelier, in his pharmaceutical laboratory at the University of Bordeaux, set out to find the secret of the wonderful tree that grows along the Atlantic coast of Canada.

In the course of his research, Masquelier, following the clues provided by footnotes in later editions of Voyages au Canada determined that the tree of which Cartier wrote was, in fact, a maritime pine tree and that a similar tree grew in abundance from Bordeaux south of the Spanish border. He was finally able to isolate the active ingredients of the pine bark and found that they conformed generally to the characteristics of the flavonoids.

In an article entitled Flavonoids and Pycnogenols

(International Journal for Vitamin and Nutritional Research 49, N3 3,307 - 311,1979) Masquelier, along with his collaborators, J. Michaud, D. La Parra, and M.C. Dumon, reported significant differences between the characteristics of his pine tree extract (which he named proanthocyanidin) and the characteristics of flavonoids. He concluded that proanthocyanidin is more properly classed as belonging to a separate and distinct class of chemicals to which we have the name "pycnogenols."

So, why is this proanthocyanidin so much better than traditional antioxidants? It is extremely bio-available, 50 times more powerful as a radical scavenger than Vitamin E, and 20 times more powerful than Vitamin C. It is totally non-toxic, and remains in the blood stream for up to 72 hours, instead of two to four hours like C and E. It even crosses the blood brain barrier. Therefore, this is the compound we use in our program, seeing dramatic results!

I also utilize antioxidant therapy on not only my detoxification patients but all my patients, especially those over 40. In fact I strongly recommend that all my patients utilize this truly amazing compound. Besides effectively dealing with an over abundant proliferation of free radicals which are generated by body toxins, I believe Pycnogenol to greatly aid in the process of detoxification, by improving and strengthening circulatory pathways. A healthy circulatory system is essential in order to effectively eliminate toxins receded deep in our body tissues. If lipophilic toxins are mobilized for elimination and circulatory pathways are diseased by age, diabetes, etc., they cannot be delivered to eliminative organs for excretion.

In fact, I believe it to be worthwhile to briefly mention some of the results I have had in my clinic and personally witnessed utilizing only this one compound.

The epidemic nature of environmental contaminants and their overwhelming damaging effects upon human health causes me to strongly recommend this antioxidant therapy whether my patients are going through the detoxification program or not. At least they can provide partial protection from future detestation to their bodies.

The following are actual case histories I have had in my office over a three month period.

Glen - Age 78
This statement date Feb. 9, 1994.

I started on Pycnogenol Dec. 20, 1993. At the time I was troubled with arthritis and respiratory disorders, a real problem to get my rest at night. After being on the product for 7 weeks it is hard to believe I could have the quality of life I have now. I rest better at night, my energy is greatly increased, pains from arthritis nearly gone, also I've been underweight all my life and I have gained 15 lbs. in the past 2 months. I will have this product in my possession and use it the rest of my life.

Kathryn

On February 8, 1994 Kathryn reported that approximately 15 children have been admitted to Dixie Medical Center with Respiratory Syncyntial Virus (RSV). This condition is usually seen in children from newborn to about five years of age, and is characterized by wide spread bronchiolar inflammatory exudate, mucosal edema, and resultant narrowing of the airway. All of these patients have some degree of hypoxemia (not enough oxygen in the blood). This condition may persist for 4-6 weeks. Kathryn also reports that she and others in her area have used Pycnogenol at 2-4 times saturation dose, given for 2-5 days to children with RSV symptoms and have had 80-90% alleviation of symptoms, usually within 8-12 hours.

Kent from - Levan, Utah

Kent reported to me that five years ago he was diagnosed with M.S. and has had severe low back pain with bad headaches this entire time. He has had to walk with a cane the entire time. Since starting on Pycnogenol, within the first few weeks his pains were gone and he is walking without his cane and this entire time he has been taking no other medications.

Robert from - St. George, Utah Age 80
(75% of men over 50 will have some degree of prostatitis)

For the past 10 to 12 years, Robert has had problems with his prostate. In 1981 he was diagnosed as being pre-cancerous. He has had painful voiding of his bladder throughout the day and 4 or 5 times per night for many years. He also reported that he had congestive heart failure and swollen extremities. After 1 month on Pycnogenol, all of these symptoms are gone, normal frequency of urination, no pains, and his heart and lungs greatly improved.

Cleo - Age 72 - Santa Clara, Utah

Diagnosed with Alzheimer's 3 or 4 years ago. This woman has been confined to a wheel chair most of the time, she can't get out of it by herself, she doesn't know her children most of the time, and doesn't know her husband died 2 years ago. She stairs blankly into space most of the time and mumbles periodically. Her daughter was given some Pycnogenol on Jan. 10th. She started her mother on a double saturation dose for 10 days then reduced it to a regular saturation dose. The daughter reports her mother is now beginning to talk to her grandchildren, gets out of her wheelchair by herself and is walking twice as good. Needless to say, she feels like it's a miracle.

Steven - Age 8

This eight year old boy from Colorado City, AZ, has had no bladder control from birth. He has wet pants and wet a bed 24 hours a day. His mother gave him 2 Pycnogenol tablets on January 23, 1994. It's been a week now and he has had maybe 2 or 3 accidents through the week, but he's a changed boy.

Brenda from - St. George, Utah

A female patient in her 30's came to my office with a history of having a simple foot surgery which had developed complications of phlebitis. Her foot and lower extremity was discolored, purplish blue, swollen and painful and she was walking on crutches. She had been having this problem for 6 weeks. She mentioned that her cardiologist was going to put her on cumadin if the problem didn't resolve soon. January 21 she began on a 120 mg dose daily and I told her to come back in a week. After 1 week the discoloration was 30% improved, swelling and pains were greatly reduced and she was walking without her crutches, her cardiologist said she wouldn't need to go on the cumadin. After 2 weeks she reported feeling 50% better.

Shay

Came into my office the other day and told me that she has had chronic bilateral shoulder pains for the past year, and she hadn't been able to sleep on either shoulder at night. She also mentioned that her right elbow had developed severe pains over the previous 2 months. After 1 week on pycnogenol, all pains were completely gone and she was sleeping comfortably.

Mary from - Nephi, Utah

Reported that she had been in a wheelchair for the past 2 1/2 years with arthritis so severe that her ankles were totally locked up. She has been in almost constant pain this entire time. After one month on pycnogenol, she is now out of her wheelchair, walking and remarkably better.

Betty

Came into my clinic on February 21, 1994 reporting that she has had diabetic neuropathy in her feet for the past seven years. She reported that her feet were completely numb from her toes to her heel. After just one day on pycnogenol she mentioned to her husband that she thought she could feel something in her feet. After one week, she reported having normal feeling in both feet. She now has to go out and buy new shoes because for the first time she realizes they have uncomfortable bumps on them.

Calvin from - St. George, Utah

This patient complained of lower back pains, when told to walk daily, he reported he hasn't been able to go for a walk in six months due to a diabetic complication of right leg thrombophelbitis. He reported pain and swelling worsened by any walking. He also reported being on cumadin for the previous six months with no response. After being on pycnogenol for two days both his pain and swelling were completely gone. He is now back to walking two miles per day without any problems.

Ellen

Came into our office to purchase Pycnogenol, and to tell us her experiences. She said that Pycnogenol is helping with her "CREST" Syndrome.

C . . . Calcium deposits of the joints
R . . . Raynaud's disease, vascular disorder of extremities.
E . . . Esophageal
S . . . Scleredema, edematous hardening of the skin
T . . . Broken blood vessels

Since being on Pycnogenol her symptoms have lessened, her hands look and feel much better and the inflammation of arthritis in her shoulder has been relieved and she now has regained full use of her right arm.

Lynn

Stated that he has had Prostrate problems and had to get up 2-3 times during the night to go to the bathroom. He had to wait to start flow. Since being on a saturation dose of Pycnogenol for 3 weeks, he said he is able to void easier, has no sudden urges to void, and usually sleeps all night.

Nicholas - age 21 from Medford, Oregon

What has come out of a little pink tablet called "pycnogenol" is a miracle.

My son, Nicholas was diagnosed when he was 14 years old with a form of Rheumatoid Arthritis. Doctor's wanted to put him on all types of steroids including liquid Gold and Prednisone which causes blindness and other severe side effects. We fought against this for years. I had him tested by the Shriners Hospital in Portland and they diagnosed him with possible Ankylosing spondelitis. He was on Azulfidine, a sulfur medication for Ankylosing Spondelitis for several years but it did not help. At 15 years of age they did surgery on the knee to remove the inflammation and to do a biopsy.

They said that this would last five years. After 3 days the swelling returned and the Rheumatoid Arthritis Specialist said that he really did not know what Nic had but they were going to call it RA anyway. They drained the knee several times after this to no avail.

Nic is now 20 years old. The RA has deteriorated hip cartilage severely and it was recommended that he have surgery in 2 years. The knee which has been 3 times its normal size since he was 14 yrs old has not had any mobility in it. Despite therapy 3 times, he has never been able to bend it. The RA went into his neck, wrist and feet causing severe pain and swelling. Nic has not been able to bend over to touch his toes, or put his shoes and socks on in over a year. His back would not bend more than a 1/4 without severe pain. His knee has been frozen in the same position - not bendable for greater than 4 years. Meclomen, an inflammatory drug has controlled the pain and some inflammation, but he continued to have a high sed rate and the swelling remained the same.

The pain and mobility is most severe in the mornings to the point that it takes over a half hour to be able to move in the morning to get ready for work. The specialist wanted Nic to be put on a new type of steroid for the rest of his life. This steroid has even more severe attributes in destroying the bodies own immune system and there is no guarantee that it would work. At the time of this writing Nic was taking 8 Meclomen a day. He said he couldn't walk, drive, or move without it. The doctor warned him that taking that large amount would cause severe damage to his major organs and even eventually kill him.

I gave Nic a bottle of Pycnogenol Friday evening, 4-22-94. I said, "promise me for my Mother's Day that you will take this faithfully." So he took two tablets - Saturday and Sunday morning. On Monday morning he took six. That morning he could bend all the way to the floor and touch his toes without any pain. He also could ben his knee over 50 degrees and felt no pain. He was able to put on his own socks and shoes for the first time in a year.

On June 10, 1994, Nic came over just beaming with delight. I noticed his new tennis shoes. "Hey, you got some new shoes! All right!" He said, "Yeah, now I can tie my own shoes, boy do they feel great on my feet."

Nic still has arthritis and what damage that has been done is done, but Pycnogenol has made things possible for this young man that he hasn't been able to do in a long time. And the rewards out weigh the disabilities. He is now taking 1 Meclomen per day. Nic is 5'5" and weighs about 110 lbs. He has very little muscle supporting his small frame. He has energy, and doesn't get tired as easily. He is starting to gain weight from building more muscle but in the beginning lost weight, (inflammation probably). He still has the arthritis but when he takes the Pycnogenol it reduces the inflammation and pain. I feel that this bio-flavonoid is a miracle. What ever it is, it is helping Nicholas walk, bend over, sleep, gain muscle control, add body weight, feeling energetic and most important not being drugged with medication and its side effects.

These few case histories should give the reader some idea of just how effective and potent this compound is. According to FDA regulations this compound is classified as a food supplement and should contain no therapeutic claims. However the research and clinical responses are very impressive and suggestive of tremendous potential in health care.

As mentioned earlier, I realized that most of the vegetables, fruits, grains, seeds, meats, fish, water, and air our bodies have been ingesting were contaminated with micro amounts of literally thousands of man-made chemicals, with known toxic effects. These micro amounts have an accumulation effect on the body, and all of which liberated an overwhelming amount of free radical oxygen molecules. Organic foods, which are foods produced without using man-made chemicals in the soil, water or air to control bugs, weeds, fungus, etc. are the foods I recommend to my patients. Organic meats are produced without the use of growth hormones, pesticides, antibiotics, etc. However, meat proteins, especially in excess are unhealthy for humans and should be avoided or used sparingly.

Contrary to popular belief, the federal government inspects less than 1% of the meat consumed in the U.S. every year. The meat that is inspected is done so by methods used to detect only a few potential chemical contaminants. At a time when our streams and oceans are badly contaminated with chemicals and waste, fish and seafood still remain the only flesh foods not required to be federally inspected.

So what can we do to help avoid polluting ourselves? Here are a few hints which you may find helpful. When eating meats, always trim fat from beef, pork and fowl because many pesticides, as in man, tend to accumulate in the animals fatty tissues. This includes trimming the skin from poultry. White meat of chicken and turkey are less fatty, therefore healthier, Pork sausage, bacon, ground beef and some deli meats are higher in fat. One should always minimize consumption of organ meat, such as liver and kidneys, because as in man, pesticides and antibiotics tend to accumulate in those filtering organs. The federal government inspection records indicate that chicken, lamb, duck, goose and rabbit contain the least amount of chemicals or drugs. You will benefit from purchasing your meats and poultry from companies who take great care to eliminate chemical residues or drugs from their products. Such companies include: Chicken from - Foster Farms of Turlock, California, Holly Farms of Wilkesboro, N.C. Turkey from - Foster Farms, Norbest of Salt Lake City. Your Beef from - Harris Ranch of California, or Hitch Enterprises, Guzman Oklahoma. Of course, in my opinion, it is best not to eat meats at all, due to the fat, cholesterol, and adverse chemical interac-

tions with the intestinal tract and body.

When preparing produce, attempt to remove poisonous surface sprays and pesticides by filling your sink with cold water. Add four tablespoons of salt and the juice of one-half of a fresh lemon. (This makes a diluted form of hydrochloric acid.) Soak fruits or vegetables 5-10 minutes, 2-3 minutes for leafy greens and 1-2 minutes for berries, i.e. strawberries - then rinse and thoroughly scrub and, whenever possible, peel vegetables and fruits. Remove outer leaves of leafy vegetables. This will help, but unfortunately won't guarantee that all pesticides will be removed because many chemicals are absorbed through the roots. More and more stores sell organically grown produce. Supply will increase as the public becomes educated and demands it. Some markets promote produce with "no detected pesticide residues" under the Nutri Clean label. Much of the produce under the Nutri Clean label has been grown organically or by farmers who are making the transition from chemical methods of pest control to biological ones. Produce with the least amount of pesticides most often include bananas, watermelon and cauliflower.

Obtaining a good source of water isn't as easy as you might think. Drinking large quantities of purified water daily acts to modify specific routes of elimination through the intestinal tract, and urinary tract. Water is considered one of the very basic nutrients of life, perhaps one of the most important! When taking into consideration all of the options available for liquid refreshment, plain old water is by far the healthiest, while a majority of other choices can actually lead to the suppression of good health.

My conclusions have been derived through clinical observation and careful study of the various research work which has been done in this field. Early on in my clinical detoxification experience, I noted that a vast majority of my patients, who were overweight, who were going through our detoxification program, were also losing weight. I also noted that these individuals also appeared to have a high success rate of keeping the weight off. I soon began to put some of the related reasons together and came to the conclusion that if anybody is desiring to lose weight, they should also be detoxifying the fatty tissues of their bodies at the same time.

If these various conclusions are valid, or even partially valid, it causes one to wonder about the 84,000,000 people in our country who are overweight, or the 34,000,000 who are obese. It also further supports the tremendous importance of proper clinical detoxification and weight loss programs.

It isn't good enough for a doctor or clinic to just say lose weight! With the extremely poor success rates in the over 4 billion dollar weight loss industry, it only seems logical that anyone mustering enough will power to change their life style and discipline themselves to eat and exercise properly should give their weight loss plan the greatest chance of success. I personally feel that weight loss without detoxification is not only going to have low success rates, but will be of risk to your health.

Detoxification combined with weight loss is unique from all other diet programs. It effectively addresses new and serious concerns about the fatty tissues of our bodies containing numerous toxic substances (fat soluble toxins), and what happens to them during weight loss. The program not only helps you effectively and safely lose weight, but it also promotes the cleansing of harmful toxins from your fatty tissues at the same time. Our program requires a new attitude about weight loss, diet and eating habits. It also requires initial strict supervision by a trained doctor in this method, which provides great support and benefit to the patient in monitoring loss of pounds, vital signs, and dealing with any complications effectively as they could arise. This type of supervision greatly increases your chances of success in reaching and maintaining your goal.

If attitudes about diet do not change amongst the general population of the United States, I fear for the future of our nations health. It is my belief that poor diet alone is responsible for a tremendously large percentage of the disease processes amongst our population. In fact one could even call the average American diet, the "disease diet".

The following eight concepts contain general rules and guidelines which any individual who desires to lose weight, must become very familiar with to succeed in our program. And again I would like to stress the point that these concepts are intended to be used permanently, from now on!!

Concept #1. Fatty foods make you fat and need to be completely eliminated from your diet. You are what you eat!! If your diet is 70% fat, your body composition will be 70% fat! According to current body rate recommendation, a male body should have 18 to 22% fat and a female body should have 23 to 27% fat ratio. Besides all of the other unhealthy risks associated with high body fat, body toxins store primarily in our fats. Therefore, I encourage keeping your fat intake down to 10% to 20%. You must learn to closely look at all labels on the foods you eat. Example: If 4 grams of fat exist for every 100 calories per serving, that food has approximately 40% fat, don't eat it! Simply add a 0 behind the fat grams to figure fat calories and divide into the calories per serving. This isn't 100% accurate, but close, and a quick way to figure it out.

Concept #2. Your attitude toward your way of eating needs to be a positive and healthy one. You must learn to enjoy eating healthy foods such as fruits, vegetables, grains, and legume's.

Concept #3. Always attempt to eat organically grown products where possible, (those free of toxic chemical residues). A call to your local markets to talk with the produce

manager will help you determine if your local stores
carry these items. As mentioned in Chapter Two, there
are a number of companies which take pride in producing organically grown foods.

Concept #4. During the first three to five weeks on the Detox
weight reduction program, meats should be eaten sparingly or totally avoided. If you feel that 80% fat meat is
something you can't do without, you should always
attempt to obtain your meats from companies which
attempt to remove all toxic contaminants when the
meats are being produced.

Concept #5. The basic recommendations for providing your
bodies with the nutrients it needs would consist of a
minimum of one or two cups of starch or three or four
slices of bread, depending upon your energy expendi-
ture, whether an office worker, (sedentary) or a construction worker, (athletic). Several of your meals
should include proteins such as beans, nuts, seeds, eggs
or fish. However, nuts and eggs are higher in fat calories, and fish runs the higher risk of toxin contamination. Calorie-dense foods exhibit the staying power
needed for heavy work or workouts, such as pastas.
Proteins are best supplied to the body by various combinations of grains and legume's, (peas, lentils, beans),
such as split pea soup with breads, rice and beans, kidney bean chili and cornbread, or baked beans with
brown bread.

Concept #6. I strongly suggest that you and or your family
make the investment in a good water filtration system
for your home. Please seek your doctor's advice when
doing so. There are literally hundreds to choose from.
Many filtration products just don't do the job. Your

doctor, if trained in the Detox program, has access to expert advise and assistance in helping you choose the right system for your needs. A mini trampoline is another recommended purchase for the program. These items are recommended to be used daily for many years to come and will produce wonderful health benefits. We often spend hundreds or even thousands of dollars on our cars yearly, but fail to realize just how important good nutrition is in keeping our bodies running properly.

Concept #7. It is very important that the health habits of good eating and exercising be maintained consistently through your life. This is not simply a one or two month program designed to quickly take the weight off, then allow you to return to the unhealthy eating and living habits. These dietary recommendations are only a small part of the detoxification program.

Concept #8. Diet however is an extremely important and vital part of being healthy. The "disease diet" will cause disease, ill health, and a diminished quality of life. I often compare eating a 40% to 90% fat diet similar to drinking large amounts of alcohol regularly, regularly taking drugs to artificially stimulate, depress, or alter body function.

It is only a matter of time before diet will be recognized as a primary factor in disease prevention or disease causation. Each individual must make that personal commitment to reduce fat intake to 20% and avoid junk. One cannot input garbage foods and expect healthy result with body function. There is no doubt that when you choose what your diet will consist of, you are literally choosing what your health will be like. It is no different than choosing to exercise or not, choosing to drink and take drugs or not, choosing to be pessimistic or optimistic. With education of the facts, you have no one to blame for your good or ill health except yourself.

By the end of 1988 and into 1990, I had officially termed my detoxification program, "Chiroholistic Detox". At this time I had quite a number of patients who had successfully gone through the program and were very pleased. It was early in 1990, when one of my patients suggested that I should teach other doctors how to do this program. The thought had never occurred, that millions of people weren't going to have access to this program or be able to find the answers to their difficult questions unless I went outside my comfortable little world of clinical practice and became more of an educator.

I also realized that this program was not just for the few, but for everyone, It is true that everyone doesn't have all of the overt signs and symptoms of bio-accumulation, however everyone is affected by the damaging effects of toxic residue in their systems and need to have this knowledge and access to detoxification.

It is now my personal belief that many of the immune suppressive disorders, reproductive disorders, nerve disorders, and many other health problems may have a direct link to toxic bio-accumulations. There is a tremendous amount of research still needed on this subject matter and associated fields. This research will not be done without proper public awareness and funding.

From 1990 to 1991, I produced a series of seminars for educating doctors and the general public. These were taught in various locations around the western U.S. in Phoenix AZ, Las Vegas NV, San Diego CA, Los Angeles CA, Salt Lake City UT, and various radio talk shows in Salt Lake City UT, Boca Rotan FL, etc. Late in 1991, I found my own practice and patients suffering (neglected), due to the splintered time schedule and splintered interests. At this time I made the choice to spend more time in the office. I personally found the greatest amount of satisfaction from private practice, helping sick people get well. My lecturing is now limited to a per invitation schedule, and quite restricted. I am hopeful that the power of the pen is mightier than the mouth, and that this book will find its' way into the hands of those who need it most.

References:
1. Williams, M., et al., "The effect of Local Temperature Changes on Sebum Excretion Rate and Forehead Surface Lipid Composition," Brit. J. of Dermatol. 88:257-262, 1973 and Root, D.E., Lionelli G.T., "Excretion of a Lipophilic Toxicant Through the Sebaceous Glands: a Case Report", J. Toxicol. Cut. & Ocular Toxicol. 6(1):13-17, 1987.
2. Wirth, A., Schlierf, G. and Schettler, G., "Physical Activity and Lipid Metabolism", Klin. Wochenschr. 57/22:1195-1201, 1979.
3. Schnare, D.W., Ben, M., Robinson, P.C., Shields, M.G., "Body Burden Reductions of PCBs, PBBs and Chlorinated Pesticides in Human Subjects", Ambio 13(5-6):378-380, 1984.
4. Root, D.E., et al, "Diagnosis and Treatment of Patients Presenting Subclinical Signs and Symptoms of Exposure of Chemicals Which Accumulate in Human Tissue", Proceedings of the National conference on Hazardous Wastes and Environmental Emergencies, May 14-16, 1985. Hazardous Materials Control Research Institute.
5. Schnare, D.W., Denk, G., Shields, M., Brunton, S., "Evaluation of a Detoxification Regimen for Fat Stored Wenobiotics", Med. Hyp. ('265-282, 1982.
6. Schnare, D.W., Robinson, P.C., "Reduction of Hexachlorobenzene and Polychlorinated Biphenyl Human Body Burdens", International Agency for Research on Cancer, Scientific Publications Series 77:597-603, 1986.

7. Occupational Health & Safety, News Digest, "Reducing Toxic Body Burdens Advancing in Innovative Technique", Vol. 2, No. 4 April 1986.

8. Kilburn, K.H. Warsaw, R.H., Shields, M.G. "Neurobehavioral Dysfunction in Firemen Exposed to polychlorinated Biphenyls 9 PCBs): Possible Improvement after Detoxification", Archives of Env. Health, Nov./Dec. 1989 [Vol. 44 (No. 6)]

9. Wisner, M.R., Shields, M., Curtis, L.D., Beckmann, S.L., "Human contamination and Detoxification: Medical Response to an Expanding Global Problem", Mab Unesco, Moscow, 1989.

10. Tretjak, Z., Shields, M., Beckmann, S.L., "PCB Reduction and Clinical Improvement by Detoxification: and Unexploited Approach?", Human & Experimental Toxicology (1990), 9, 235-244.

11. Wolff, M.S., Anderson, H.A., Selikoff, I.J., "Human Tissue Burdens of Aromatic Chemicals in Michigan, J.A.M.A. 247:2112-2116, 1982.

Chapter Three

REAL PEOPLE WHO
ARE GETTING BETTER

(five actual case histories)

Some of the names of patients have been changed to protect patient / doctor confidentiality. However, actual histories and rates of recovery were used in every case.

Patient #1.

Sallie was a 41 year old female, who I came to eventually know as an intelligent, kind, articulate, and friendly person, who enjoyed teaching violin lessons and writing articles for magazines. However, when Sallie first came to our clinic, she was quite a different person.

When I had my first consultation with Sallie, she appeared disoriented, confused, couldn't concentrate or carry on a conversation, and appeared quite depressed. On that first visit, when I explained to her how much effort it was going to take on her part, time commitment, and consistency, she changed her mind several times about going through the detoxification regimen. After some reassurance from me, she finally decided to give it her best shot. After all, she had been suffering with this problem for many years, and had tried a number of unsuccessful treatments, diet plans, etc. Sallie had been referred to my office by another doctor who believed she may benefit from a course of clinical detoxification.

The referring doctor noted a complex set of symptoms resembling both Candida and Pre-menstrual Syndrome. She initially complained of sever head pains, moderate to severe constipation which required regular enemas, a great deal of severe mental confusion, snowy vision, extreme severe fatigue and depression which were both worsened by PMS intervals. Sallie also initially complained of moderate dizziness and indigestion, mild stomach pains and back pains. She reported moderate to severe reoccurring flu-like symptoms, allergies, and memory loss. She complained of severe eye irritations, and irritability.

As mentioned in earlier chapters, when most doctors hear a report of this array of symptoms, they think of various mental problems such as depression, psychosomatic and mental disfunction. Millions of such cases would normally be referred to a psychologist for analyzing and the use of various drugs to help with depression or the stabilization of mood swings. Most medical doctors or clinical psychologists are not familiar with the related affects of bio-accumulations or Multiple Chemical Sensitivity, MCS. They may not even consider this as a clinical possibility. Therefore they wrongly refer their patients for mental help, however well meaning it may be. Now, I am in no way saying that all patients with this set of symptoms have bio-accumulation, or would benefit from clinical detoxification, however, I am saying these patients should be considered for a consultation with a doctor trained in clinical detoxification.

Sallie mentioned that previous medical treatments for some of these conditions had been, two rounds of full spectrum antibiotics which gave no relief and aggravated her condition. I spent quite some time educating Sallie about the many aspects of toxic accumulations on the body, what they do to our bodies and how to rid the system of these toxins. I believe that patient education is as important as the actual therapy. I have learned over the years that patient compliance requires more than simple trust in the doctor; it requires a basic understanding of the clinical condition and the methods of treatment. Therefore, patient education is essential to a successful treatment program in which the patient is motivated to be compliant with recommendations.

Sallie in her own words wrote the following critique of our program: "At the time I was referred to Dr. Hobson, I was suffering from severe head pains, I thought to be sinus related; constipation to the point of needing regular enemas; a great deal of mental confusion; snowy vision; extreme fatigue and depression, usually relating to premenstrual.

The medical treatment for this condition was two rounds of full spectrum antibiotics which gave no relief and aggravated my condition. My symptoms paralleled those of candida. After relating such to another doctor, he, knowing of Dr. Hobsons' work, referred me to him. Dr. Hobson took a great deal of time educating me to the program in my initial visit. He was professional in his approach. I felt I was in good hands.

Within the first week I noticed immediate improvement. The depression was lifted and the head pain was greatly reduced. Within two and one-half weeks, constipation cleared up. Skin eruptions were greatly reduced and healing.

I believe this treatment to be of great worth and of benefit to most people in clearing up disorders and regulating bodily functions." (end of critique)

After approximately six weeks of consistent effort and daily compliance to the detoxification regimen, Sallie had made tremendous improvement. She reported feeling 100% better, having no symptoms of head pains, indigestion, stomach pains, constipation, fatigue, flu like symptoms, skin rash, allergies, tiredness, and irritability. She also reported feeling 80% to 90% improved with dizziness, mental confusion, and memory. All of her PMS symptoms were gone. She truly was a different person than the one I witnessed just six weeks earlier. Sallie said, "I feel like I have my old self back, and I can now do all of the things that I have been wanting to do for a long time and couldn't."

Patient #2

This patient was a 39 year old female named Jeneane, who was referred to my office by another doctor. She appeared tired, underweight, and had many of the symptoms associated with toxic bio-accumulations. During her initial history Jeneane reported an exposure to chlorine gas in Las Vegas, NV several years earlier which started most of her symptoms. She reported that whenever she was around a pool from that time until now, she became very ill. She reported a general weakness in her lungs which caused them to have, in her own words, "a burning, achy, hurt feeling, and constriction around her throat." Jeneane also reported that she regularly had her house sprayed, monthly, for bugs.

On Jeneane's initial visit she reported her symptoms on a regular basis as follows: severe head pains, fatigue, flu like symptoms, allergies, tiredness, mental confusion, memory loss, and irritability. Also, moderate recurring symptoms of insomnia, dizziness, indigestion, and eye irritations. And Janeane also reported mild symptoms of vomiting, stomach pains, back pains, and skin rash.

Jeneane followed the detoxification regimen with a consistency of 95%. After approximately five weeks, Jeneane had made very good progress. She then reported her symptom level as follows: Flu like symptoms, mental confusion, insomnia, eye irritations, indigestion, vomiting, back pains, stomach pains, and skin rashes all 100% improved. Also her head pains, fatigue, allergies, dizziness, and memory loss all 90% improved.

Patient #3

This 46 year old female, named Ranae, came to my office as a histological technician who worked in a hospital lab. She had numerous somatic complaints and reported that she had been taking serum injections for allergies for about three months with out any results. She had previously been diagnosed by an eye, ear, nose, and throat specialist as having irreparable damage or burns to the mucous membrane linings of her nose and sinuses. This condition left her highly susceptible to many upper respiratory and sinus infections. She also exhibited many bio-accumulation symptoms such as: severe head pains, flu like symptoms, eye irritations, skin rash, allergies, tiredness, and irritability. Also moderate symptoms of insomnia, dizziness, stomach pains, back pains and constipation.

Ranae had six children, was single, and found it necessary to work full time as many women do these days. However, due to the numerous health complaints, she found it increasingly difficult to care for her kids, her job, or herself.

Needless to say, Ranae was a definite candidate for clinical detoxification. After three weeks on the program, Ranae reported that she had just seen her E.E.N.T. doctor, (eye, ear, nose and throat), who was very impressed with her progress. He told Ranae that it appeared that the mucous lining of her nose was beginning to run again and produce mucous, which usually wouldn't be considered good, however, in Ranae's case it was. She had not had a runny nose since she was first diagnosed with damaged or burned mucous membrane linings. The E.E.N.T. doctor also told Ranae that whatever she had been doing, to keep it up!

Ranae's therapy program lasted longer than originally anticipated due to the chronic severity of the condition, and her inability to maintain consistency with the detoxification protocol. Raising six kids, on her own, and working full time is plenty of excuse I felt. Anyway, after approximately 10 weeks,

Ranae's symptom picture had made some very good improvements. Her head, flu like symptoms, eye irritations and insomnia had all improved by at least 50%. Her skin rashes improved 60%, Irritability improved 80%, back pains 90%, and dizziness, indigestion, constipation, mental confusion, and memory loss improved 100%. Ranae reported having much more energy and could do so much more with the time she had.

Patient #4

This was a 50 year old male named Curtis. Curtis came to my office from Texas having been diagnosed with Multiple Chemical Sensitivity by Dr. William Rae M.D. of Texas and suppressed immune system function by Dr. Alan Levin M.D. of California. This condition had been affecting Curtis for over 20 years.

Curtis had tried moving to several locations over the years to see if it would help his condition. He had been told by several previous doctors that he would probably need to move from a large city environment to that of a small town, due to the amount of air and water pollution in the big cities. Curtis was a computer programmer and program writer working for Chevron Oil Company in Houston when he decided to move. He reported that his abilities to concentrate and do his job effectively were slowly deteriorating over the previous several years. He found it necessary to use a filtration mask when outside, drive with an air scrubber while in his car, use water and air filtration devices in his home.

Curtis had been the primary income provider for his wife and seven children, and he was reluctant to leave his great job in Houston. However, due to deteriorating health he was more or less forced to. Curtis had also been previously diagnosed with Vasculitis, heart rhythm disorders, Hashemoto's Thyroiditis. He was taking medications of synthroid, calan, lanoxin for these various health complaints.

Curtis also had an interesting health history in that his cousins, twin sisters, and father all had similar symptoms and diagnosis. This finding always causes any practitioner to theorize about genetic predisposition verses common environmental contamination. I suspect a combination of both is the more plausible association.

Curtis's appearance and demeanor were similar to other MCS patients I had seen before. However, he had a much more chronic and lengthy history than most of my previous patients. He was underweight, frail in appearance, his speech was somewhat disorganized, and he had a difficult time concentrating. He had numerous complaints consistent with bio-accumulation such as: headaches, dizziness, fatigue, skin rash, tiredness, mental confusion, memory loss and irritability.

I anticipated from the onset that Curtis' treatment time was going to be somewhat prolonged, and that his body needed more time than the average to heal. You'll recall from previous chapters, that bio-accumulation damages the nervous, reproductive, and immune systems, allowing the patient to fall susceptible to various disease processes. The goal in Curtis' case was to eliminate the offending toxins, eliminate additional contamination, and allow his body to begin healing itself if possible. I believe that in most cases, if the doctor can accurately find the real cause of the problem and eliminate it, the body will then be allowed to begin healing.

Curtis underwent an intensive eight week course of detoxification therapy with good but slow results. After approximately eight weeks he reported feeling 50% better. After this intensive care period, Curtis underwent a less intense period of therapy which required a daily regimen of detox baths, rebounding, strict diet, and taking of recommended nutrients for an additional three months. At this point, he reported feeling 60% to 70% improved.

For the next eight months, Curtis came into the office once

every week to ten days for evaluation and treatment when necessary. After approximately 14 months he reported feeling 80% improved. He could now go to grocery stores, church, and ball games without getting sick. He could travel, eat some non-organic foods and drive downtown without getting sick. His weight had gone from 125 lbs. to 153 lbs. He now could concentrate long enough to work at his computer, write letters and carry on a conversation with a group of people without falling apart emotionally. Just about all of his initial symptoms were clearing well except mild irritability and fatigue.

Curtis recently made an appeal for disability assistant to a state agency, which allowed an opportunity to obtain the following history in his own words.

"I last performed gainful employment in December, 1991, while working for Chevron in Houston, Texas. After receiving competent medical advice on the long term nature of my illness, which included a prognosis for extensive therapy, an extended recovery period, and long term limitations on lifestyle, I entered chemical detoxification therapy in March, 1992. I have continued this therapy on a daily basis for over 16 months with gradual, and now recently, accelerated indications of improvement. Only recently have I optimistically viewed a return to gainful employment as a distinct possibility.

To achieve these results, I have worked faithfully and hard! During the last 16 months I estimate I have expended almost 1500 hours in direct therapy. In addition to the direct therapy, several hours of each day of therapy have always been 'recovery hours' after each session ends. These are hours where I am mentally and physically impaired from the therapy itself. This impairment period results from the mobilization of toxins during the chemical detoxification process.

My illness has impacted my entire life. Initial symptoms were recurrent lymph infections by age 4, slow physical development, and unexplained heart palpitations by late teens. As the illness progressed, I also began to have periods of overwhelming fatigue, especially following meals and within certain buildings and other closed environments. Later, following periods of outdoor air pollution, I developed flu like illness and then chronic sinus and sore throat infections. Daily muscle and joint aches became common. Through time, allergies to almost all foods gradually developed, accompanied by weight loss from 150 lbs. to less than 110 lbs. A condition similar to irritable bowel syndrome followed. Gradually, I could no longer eat any foods except organically grown foods. Subsequently any airborne pollution such as the slightest exposure to automobile exhausts, soaps, insecticides, paint, ink, cologne, or perfume impaired me both psychologically and cognitively.

Repeated attempts to find assistance through medical professionals failed until about 8 years ago. Through my own life experience I had come to understand the problem as an immune disorder, and from readings encountered in Graduate School, I knew of a team of physicians in San Francisco who were treating the illness. To gain their assistance, I lived away from my family, who were in Utah, for over a year, and concurrently gained employment with San Francisco based Chevron. These physicians identified the immune disorder calling it Environmental Illness, and proposed that my auto-immune condition, a thyroid disease, and my irregular heart patterns were conditions associated with the illness. Perhaps their greatest assistance to me, in addition to the direct treatment of the thyroid and heart components, was their education on how to live and cope with chronic immune disfunction.

This education included both short term advice on how to modify a person's stress on the immune system as well as the long term effects of bioaccumulation. As explained to me, bioaccumulation of toxic chemicals would gradually occur for me within my body organs, brain, and fatty tissues. An initial proposal by Dr. Saiffer, herself having Environmental Illness, was that my condition had already deteriorated to the point where detoxification therapy, either immediately, or in the future, was unavoidable. She urged detoxification therapy provided by Dr. Rea in Dallas, although at that time in 1985, the program was not well developed nor was the process well understood. Through the team efforts of Dr. Levin, Dr. Becker, and Dr. Weinreb in San Francisco. I was able to adapt to my immune disorder well enough to maintain employment for 7 more years.

Repeated attempts to gain medical insurance benefits for detoxification, or even recognition of the illness, prevented me from obtaining this therapy. Even in 1992, when my long term disability was unavoidable, Chevron's insurance carrier would not recognize environmental illness nor approve detoxification therapy. Today the therapy is still viewed as experimental by the insurance industry, and of course, very expensive and long term. Recently medical findings in breast cancer research, and the suspected link to the bioaccumulation of toxins, will likely advance the science of detoxification and validation of therapy for insurance purposes.

Recently, the National Center for Disease Control has re-labeled Environmental Illness more descriptively as Chronic Fatigue Immune Disfunction Syndrome, or CFIDS.

In 1989, Chevron transferred me from San Francisco to Houston. Several months before my actual disability started in 1991, I traveled from Houston to Dallas to see Dr. Rea. At that time my illness had progressed to the point where I was having chronic mental disfunction. He counseled that a serious non-reversible condition, called Toxic Brain Syndrome may be developing, as well as a complete immunological breakdown which could lead to long term hospitalization. The blood plasma tests from that visit concluded that I had concentrations of toxic chemicals that were several times higher than clients already ill with Environmental Illness. Ultimately, without insurance coverage, or the realistic ability of our family of 9 to pay directly for therapy, Dr. Rea made several suggestions which eventually precipitated our family move from our urban environment in Texas to our more rural environment in southern Utah. Dr. Michael Hobson, a St. George Chiropractor, and director to the National Detoxification Institute, provided us an alternative treatment approach for just a fraction of the cost.

The results of the detoxification therapy for 16 months has been very rewarding to me. The following types of gains have been made:

1. About 2-4 months into the therapy, my general level of fatigue decreased to the point where I was not exhausted by just being on my feet.

2. About 6 months into the therapy, I was able to reduce my heart medication by half.

3. By 8 months I was able to go into food stores briefly and not become mentally confused.

4. By 9 months, I began to notice that if I stopped the detoxification therapy for at least 2 days, my psychological state cleared, and capacity to communicate increased, so that I was able to write letters. I had not written letters for months.

5. By 10 months the awareness that I could do some driving again in traffic without becoming irritable and confused by exhaust emissions.

6. Six months ago sensitivity to hair sprays, perfumes, and colognes decreased to a level where I was able to have increasing contact with Church functions each Sunday morning.

7. Within the last 4 months I was able to start eating a few non-organic foods without having disabling mental and physical reactions. Two months ago I was able to have an entire meal of non-organic food. Last month I was able to eat at a restaurant with my family!

8. Recently, the desire to read and cognitive ability to remember what I've read.

Although these gains have been made, I am hopeful some other critical components of wellness will return to me. These might include:

1.   A lack of toxicity to inks and paper. I still cannot touch newspapers and magazines through skin contact, or breathing, without adverse reactions.
2.   Ability to eat processed foods which may have preservatives or additives.
3.   Ability to be in stores, homes, or other places where newly made products such as plastics, carpets, paints, or building products have been used.
4.   Improvement in mental functioning, including short term memory gains, lack of confusion, and indecisiveness following any exposure to chemicals.
5.   Psychological and spiritual recovery from extreme irritability, despair, and depression when fatigued or following exposure to chemicals.
6.   A return of aspects of intelligence which have been lost - specifically the ability to mentally plan, visualize, and synthesize information. Currently I am still frustrated at trying to accomplish most mental tasks even when feeling 'well'. Writing this appeal has been a major achievement for me.

As a family, we have made countless adjustments to my disability. My wife has temporarily assumed the role of wage earner and I the homemaker, although with my improvement, we now believe a future readjustment will be made. Major home modifications have been made to lower any toxicity factors including removal of all carpeting and drapes, use of ceramic floor tile through the whole home, and a conversion from gas to electric heat.

We have removed all but essential books from our home and magazines or newspapers are kept in sealed cabinets. We have to avoid the use of any pesticides, use of perfumes and control the use of soaps. Outdoor application only of hair sprays was mandatory. Until recently, all my meals had to be meticulously prepared from totally organic foods. Organic foods had to be purchased from special stores in Las Vegas and Salt Lake City. Purifying air filters have been used in my bedroom and in the automobile.

The detoxification therapy is a daily home-based activity which requires approximately 3 hours for me to complete. Some days the therapy is done twice. Each therapy session involves the mobilization of body toxins from body tissues into the blood stream using aerobic exercise, elevation of body temperature through hot water baths, and oral administration of nicotinic acid. Large quantities of pure water are consumed and care is taken to replace lost minerals and vitamins. During the first weeks of therapy, my mental condition would dramatically worsen during each therapy session and continue sympathetically for several days before 'clearing'. Most noticeably to me were long periods of depression, irritability, and diminished ability to mentally function. Recent sessions are producing only 6-9 hours of impairment and with less intensity of symptoms.

Due to the gradual, but still continuing recovery, it is important to me that the detox therapy remain a part of my daily life. Weekly experiences with exposures to environmental conditions both reward me with the confidence that things are gradually getting better, but also with the understanding that the gains are still fragile." (end of Curtis' personal statement)

I anticipate that Curtis will continue to slowly progress back to a "normal" symptom level. However, he should expect a permanent susceptibility to a heavy dose of chemicals in air, water, and food. In my opinion, the longer he goes without heavy contamination, and maintains his detox daily protocol, he should get stronger and stronger.

Patient #5

This patient was a 57 year old female named Vickie. Vickie came to my office referred from another detoxification patient who we treated successfully who had MS. Vickie complained of a multitude of vague but moderate symptoms such as: head pains, back pains, fatigue, skin rash, tiredness, mental confusion, memory loss and irritability.

Vickie's primary complaints were daily fatigue which effected her quality of life such that she just couldn't enjoy her daily existence. She felt that her mental abilities were also diminished, feeling like she was in a fog all of the time. She reported that she had not had these symptoms for more than 18 months.

Vickie responded quite well. After approximately three weeks she reported feeling 90% improved. She just couldn't believe that she could feel so much better so fast. I told her that one thing in her favor was the amount of time that she had had the symptoms, only 18 months. After four weeks Vickie felt 100% improved and ready for the maintenance program. At this point she was asked to continue eating like I had taught her, continue exercising daily and go through the detox cycle one or two times per month, and schedule with our office one check up every three months.

Thus far, she has maintained very well.

Chapter Four

METHODS BY WHICH LIPOPHILIC TOXINS ARE CLEANSED FROM THE FATS

The various methods were previously discussed in chapter two, "The development of the Chiroholistic Detox program" with some detail, however this chapter will discuss some of the other details not mentioned.

You must remember that the basic detox cycle is not very complex. However, without the specific combination of the various methods, the effective cleansing of toxins from the fats will not occur. Also, as mentioned earlier, the information in this book is not designed to train the untrained to administer the program. There are many possible complications and variations that may occur among different people, during a treatment program. These complications need to be effectively handled by a doctor trained in this method of detoxification.

A brief overview of the treatment program consists of the following: one to three detox cycles per day, eating organically with primarily vegetarian foods, drinking purified water - one gal. per day, and take steps to live in a clean uncontaminated house. As chapter two indicates, the detox cycle consists of simply 30 minutes rebounding exercise primarily to create a positive/negative "G" force jumping up and down and taking specific doses of B3. Immediately after jumping on the mini-trampoline, take a shower to cleanse the skin of any dirt, oils, etc., then into the detox bath for 20 minutes. Also, taking daily prescribed supplements are included. We continue to prescribe 5 to 20 minutes sunbathing for most individuals for therapeutic effects of the sun on the skin.

The detox cycle is designed to first mobilize stored fat toxins, deliver them to the circulatory system, then modify all of the natural routes of elimination. These routes include the digestive system with diet, perspiratory system with heat, and urinary system with increased fluid intake. These various cleansing body systems are assisted by the taking of specific supplements to restore essential minerals lost during the program. Also, these specialized nutrients are designed to bind toxins from the intestinal tract for elimination. Also, specific substances are added to the detox bath water to assist the detoxification through the skin.

Over the years of administering the detox program to all shapes, sizes and ages of people, I have discovered that with proper modifications just about anyone can go through the program. You don't need to be in great shape or be an athlete, you just need the desire to work with the doctor administering the program. Often I begin the program with the client only jumping two to five minutes per day, with a balance bar, before the detox bath. The detox bath may have to be 90 to 102 degrees to begin with if problems with heat are present.

For the past eight years, our programs have been offered as an outpatient service only. Our patients have been taught how to perform their detox baths and exercises at home. However due to the growing interest, the National Detoxification Institute is currently in the planning and development stages of opening a larger facility to provide living, eating, and treatment facilities, on an in house basis. Wherein individuals wishing to come for this treatment can stay for one to six weeks at a time. Opening should occur in the fall of 1994.

In chapter one page twenty-six, you read about a study by Ashford in 1984 where he discussed bio-accumulations affecting different people differently according to personal habits, living environment, genetic background, etc. I have also found that the amount of time someone is exposed to a toxin has an effect on damage done and speed of healing. For example, I would expect to see a patient working in a chemical factory for 20 years in a big city more effected, with more damage to their nervous, immune, and reproductive systems.

Also their tissues would be heavily loaded with toxic accumulates. The detoxification program does have its limitations. It will only remove the poisons so fast, and it cannot restore permanently damaged organs to healthy function. Over time, once the toxins have been removed, the bodies miraculous, innate healing abilities will begin healing. I believe that immune system function can improve, nervous system can improve and damaged reproductive systems can become stronger.

Too often in health care, accurate diagnosis, finding the true cause of the problem, is missed. Medications are prescribed to only control the symptoms without ever treating the cause of the problem. In such cases, the best you can hope for is temporary relief of symptoms, not a cure. This is unfortunate, and causes many billions of wasted health care dollars yearly in the United States. I strongly believe that detoxification is necessary for everyone and that a major portion of many of our country's (and any industrial developed country's) health care needs are associated with toxic accumulations of the body.

Preventative health care is supposedly the wave of the future. Many American hospitals are beginning to provide services for disease prevention, prescribing exercise, good nutrition, and a healthy attitude. This is a good step in the right direction, however only a partial step. Because of my profession, I have a different viewpoint of modern, American medicine. I believe that prescription pharmaceuticals, are vastly over utilized. I also believe that the major corporations who produce, market and sell these drugs are extremely powerful in government, and in our private health care delivery system.

It is unfortunate that any organization or group can have such power over what is supposedly a non-bias, caring, healing profession who objectively examines, diagnoses, and prescribes therapy for their ill patients. All to often I have witnessed the abuse of prescribed pain killers, muscle relaxers, sleeping medications, drugs to control excessive acid in the stomach, and anti-depressants, etc.

For example, I have had numerous patients come to me with head, or back pains. Quite often these patients have experienced these problems for months and even years without ever being properly examined, diagnosed, or prescribed proper therapy. Is this because their previous doctors are bad, or not caring? No! I am not suggesting anything like that. I am saying that if the health care professional doesn't recognize the problem, they will often say, "we're not sure what's causing the problem" or "this is just tension, take this drug to ease your pain symptoms." This all too common approach, is often just treating the symptoms, not the problem. It appears that the pharmaceutical companies would have us believe that symptom treatment is adequate medical care. This attitude is very inadequate. Covering the symptom therapy, not only prolongs or inhibits the seeking of good health care, but often causes more damage that could have been prevented with appropriate care.

I am not totally down on our country's pharmaceutical companies. There are needed and helpful medications that improve quality of life, prolong life and are necessary. I am totally down on the over utilization of medications that just mask symptoms and lull both doctor and patient into thinking adequate therapy is being accomplished.

I have witnessed, thousands of times in my own clinical practice, back or head pain patients who have been told there was nothing that could be done for their pains. Then after appropriate examination, finding mechanical disfunction of the spinal column which was causing aggravation in both joint and nerve. After appropriate rehabilitation of the offending mechanical spinal problem, not only did the symptoms leave permanently, but other nerve functional problems also cleared. Yet these clients had been taking pain medications for years for these conditions. This is but a small example of the doctors misunderstanding the causative factors of disease, mis-diagnosis and inappropriate care given.

To render true preventative medicine, the doctor needs to truly understand the underlying cause of the disease or symptom. I believe that health care in the United States would advance tremendously if doctors would stop to ask, "why does this patient get so many colds", or "if the pain killers only temporarily diminish the pain, yet the patient continues to suffer, could I be missing the true cause of this condition." Often because of pride, or ignorance, the doctor fails to admit that he or she could be missing something. Often the patient is simply, and falsely told that, "nothing can be done for your suffering."

If health care learns to treat the potential problem before the damage to the human body begins, true preventative medicine will have been rendered. If all health care providers regularly counsel their patients in the habits causing ill health, preventative medicine will begin to prevail. There are those in the sales end, (marketing), of the pharmaceutical companies that wouldn't like these concepts at all!

If health care providers in the U.S. understood the severity of bioaccumulation, its cause, and effect, they would readily prescribe this therapy for the potential prevention for numerous related disease conditions.

Everyone, patient and doctor alike, needs to only stop and ask themselves some simple questions like: "How many disease processes are associated with suppressed immune system function?" If you don't know, perhaps you would be shocked to find that a very large percentage, perhaps majority, of disease processes are related to weak immune system function. Another interesting question a research team should ask is,

"How does the immune system treat a cell or tissue loaded with lipophilic toxic residues, or would it attack such a tissue?" Or one may ask, "How many diseases are associated with damaged nervous system function? How many mental disorders are caused by organic damage from chemicals. When the brain is contaminated with toxic residues, what symptoms will it cause?" When one truly understands the scope of this problem, it quickly becomes evident that it is a major player in the arena of causative factors for disease in our country.

Any treatment program that reduces damage to the immune system or can help improve immune system function is extremely important and necessary.

One of the attractive points of the clinical detoxification program is that it is very safe. A vast majority of individuals can go through the program without complication. It provides great incentive and hope for the overweight individuals. Contraindications, reasons for not doing the program, are few. In most cases, our program can be modified to work with just about anybody.

Chapter Five

APPLICATION OF EDUCATION, KEY TO HEALING

In chapter one, I posed the question, to myself, "Why are these people getting sick, and why are they getting better with this treatment?" This same question, I hope you can answer! I now realize that some narrow minded health care practitioners might say it's purely faith. Some might sat it's simply psychosomatic, or all in their heads! There will always be the "doubting Thomases" in this world.

My opinion is that a majority of doctors are doing a great service, helping their patients, and doing their best. Doctors are only human, they do make mistakes, and when a statement is said like, "this is all in your head" I believe that this stems from mostly ignorance of the facts. However the facts are clear, patients recoveries are real. It's virtually impossible for any one doctor to know everything about health care, good or bad. And if any of us think we do, we have lost our objectivity and our quality of service.

When asked how I would judge recovery or improvement, I say if the patients symptoms clear up, their suffering dissipates, normal function is restored to their lives, they are recovering! A true healer or doctor, is primarily interested in alleviating the suffering of humanity, to restore the quality of life to their patients. I have no doubt in my own mind that toxic accumulations in the human body cause tremendous damage and suffering to the human body. I also have no doubt that systemic cleansing of lipophilic toxins is perhaps one of the most important treatments of our day and age.

You will recall in chapter 3, patient #3 named Ranae, had had symptoms similar to Candida, Pre-Menstrual Syndrome, and numerous infections. She had been diagnosed with all these conditions by various doctors. I have no doubt that she actually had these various conditions, however, the question had never been asked what was causing these problems. The doctor who referred her to me suspected suppressed immune system function. It is important to note that Ranae had been treated by various over the counter (OTC) and prescription medications for a number of years for these conditions. She had also tried various diets all of which, including the medications, provided only temporary relief.

Ranae could have easily been told, "You're going to have to learn how to live with this", or "There is nothing we can do for this", or "Just take these medications to help relieve the symptoms." Many thousands of individuals suffering like Ranae, are told these same things. Thousands never really find the true answer as to why they have these problems. Thousands concede, every year to the notion that they will forever live with these pains and problems and that symptomatic medications are the best that can be done.

Ranae is glad that she didn't accept mediocre health care, that she continued to look for answers. She no longer has these symptoms, or conditions. Her immune system is healthier, stronger functioning, more efficient without the burden of toxic residues continually suppressing and destroying it.

Currently, the accumulation of toxic residues in human fatty tissues, is mostly unrecognized as a cause of disease. The current facts on this disorder have all the markings of a national epidemic, even a world epidemic of industrialized countries. If left unrecognized by health care providers, millions will needlessly suffer over the next decade. Again, I strongly believe millions of suffering people can be helped with this knowledge. Billions of health care dollars may be saved by preventing the damage done by toxins to the human body.

I am hopeful that the following information has been gleaned by the reader at this point:

Fact #1:   All persons living in the U.S. have toxic bioaccumulates in their bodies.

Fact #2:   These toxic bioaccumulates are slowly destroying your immune, nervous, and reproductive systems.

Fact #3:   These toxins unavoidably enter our bodies through the air, water, and foods we eat.

Fact #4:   Toxins that are the most damaging are lipophilic (toxins that attract to and stay in the body fats). They will not leave the body without proper detoxification technique.

Fact #5:   A damaged immune system will cause numerous secondary infections and diseases in the human body. Damaged nervous and reproductive systems will also lead to numerous secondary problems associated with those systems.

Fact #6:   Clinically researched techniques for cleansing the lipophilic toxins are available and are successfully helping those who know where to get help.

If you didn't understand these facts, re-read chapters one and two. Fact five is one that requires much thought! Any practitioner should always ask, "What is the real cause of my patients symptoms?" Too often medications are prescribed to alleviate symptoms without ever considering the cause. Medications may very well help reduce the symptoms. However, if cause isn't properly treated, cure will never come. Addiction to medication may occur. If this book does anything, I hope it will stimulate additional thought as to potential cause of the numerous health complaints seen millions of times daily in the U.S. I hope that both patients and doctors will seriously consider this possibility.

You can know all the secrets of the universe, however if you don't properly apply this knowledge, you might as well have never learned this knowledge. It can only make you a fool.

Often I have seen wonderful results and healing take place, and conditions disappear with our treatment program, only to find that two months, or one year later the patient has gone back to their old ways, and relapsed. This is very frustrating to say the least. Health is not the responsibility of the doctors! Those who think this way will always find good health an illusive thing. Every individual must take responsibility and action to improve and maintain their own good health. Healthy life styles produce good health, unhealthy life styles produce ill health. It's not always quite that simple, however. Most doctors are now beginning to realize just how important preventative medicine is. There really isn't any magic pill to make you healthy, or any outside force. Good health must come from within, a commitment to living healthy. If you think, I just can't do that, you're probably right, and you shouldn't expect to be healthy.

The techniques learned during the Chiroholistic Detox program are essentials for preventative medicine. They are principles, which if followed, will serve you well through the rest of your life. Every patient who has gone through my program is strongly counseled to continue practicing healthy living habits learned during the program. It isn't that difficult to understand that if one goes back to life styles that caused their ill health, they will again become ill!

Habits are extremely difficult to alter. Bad habits are hard to break, new habits are difficult to establish. I often have told mothers going through our program that changing their families eating habits now may seem difficult, but they may very well be changing and improving their families health for a life time or even generations to come. For example the American diet is one that is now changing due to an increasing awareness of fats, cholesterol, salt, fiber, excessive sugars, etc. Americans are finally beginning to realize that generations of bad eating habits were wrong, leading to heart disease, colon disease, and numerous other degenerative disorders associated with bad eating habits. The detox program throws in a few new wrinkles to the equation.

Therefore, regaining your good health will take more than just going through a one month treatment program. This goal must begin with the realization that commitment to new habits and the discarding of some old habits will be a lifetime one. This commitment must be motivated by knowledge and sincere desire. Insufficient motivation or desire leads to failure, which we humans all do regularly. However, if you have that success attitude, of continual effort and improvement, you can obtain and maintain this goal of good health.

You can also become a healer or provider of knowledge to family and loved ones. Who would gain pertinent knowledge to life and health preservation and not share it with someone they also want to be healthy and happy? There is strength in numbers, a committed group will often succeed easier than an individual.

Another important point to remember is that at the completion of the detoxification program, patients often feel 90 to 100% improved, or have less symptoms. Symptoms are the things that originally brought the patient seeking help. However, in most cases, symptoms are just the tip of the iceberg, so to speak. Often, major problems may have been there for years, not causing symptoms, yet greatly effecting your health. Tissues will often need to be aggravated for many years before becoming disfunctional or diseased, and begin producing symptoms. One should never assume that if they are not feeling any symptoms that they do not need to take safeguards to protect their good health!

This has been one of the worst attitudes among the American population, which has persisted for decades, that must be changed if we are to ever come up in our health index, as mentioned earlier. Health does not come from a magic pill or potion, or from anything without. It comes from within, healthy living habits and application of your knowledge of preventative medicine.

I hope that the reader can glean some helpful information from the reading of this book. I hope that any knowledge gained will be put to appropriate use and a development of a desire for greater health. I hope that you, the reader, will take the time to investigate further, to see if this method could help you. I know it can.

Index

Alzheimer's 34, 39

benzene 9
bioaccumulation 1, 13, 23, 49, 56, 59

cancer 7, 8, 16, 23, 34
candida albicans 4, 54, 55, 74
carbon monoxide 14, 18
carcinogens 6
chiroholistic detoxification program 31, 49, 67, 76
chloracne, 8
chlordane 15, 20, 21
chlorobenzene 9
chronic fatigue 3, 26, 56, 61, 66
contamination 10, 13, 21
CREST syndrome 42

DDE 9, 34
detox bath 33, 67
detoxification program 31, 32, 34, 44, 54, 57, 60, 69, 77
diazinon 16, 21
disfunctions, liver 7

ebstein barr 4
ethylbenzene 9
ethylene 10
ethylphenol 8

free radical 24, 25, 34, 43

head pains 3, 16, 20, 26, 55, 66
heart attach 34
heptachlor 16
herbicides 28
HpCDD 9
HxCDD 9
hydrochloric acid 44
hydrochloric acid 44
hyperthermia 31

lipophilic toxins 32, 33, 67, 73, 75
liver disorders 34

mononucleosis 4

Multiple Chemical Sensitivity 11, 27, 32, 54, 58
musculoskeletal pains 3, 26

National Human Adipose Tissue Survey 5, 27
nutri clean label 44
nutri clean label 44

OCDD 8

Parkinson's 34
PeCDD 9
pesticide 10
pesticide toxicology 12, 13, 43, 44
phlebitis 34, 40, 41
pollutants (indoor) 14
polychlorinated biphenyls 6
polychlorinated dibenzofurans 7
polynuclear aromatic hydrocarbons 13
pre-menstrual syndrome 54, 55
psychosomatic 4, 73
pyenogenols 37, 38, 39, 40, 41, 42
pyenogenols 37, 38, 39, 40, 41, 42

respiratory syncyntial virus (RSV) 38
respiratory syncyntial virus (RSV) 38

sarcoma cancer 16
scurvey 35
skin disorders 3
stroke 34
styrene 8

toluene 9
toxins 5, 20

vitamin c 34, 37
vitamin e 34, 37

weight loss 45, 46
weight loss 45, 46

xylene 8